Published in Great Britain by
L.R. Price Publications Ltd, 2021
27 Old Gloucester Street,
London, WC1N 3AX
www.lrpricepublications.com

Cover artwork by L.R. Price Publications Ltd
Copyright © 2021

ISBN-13: 9781838061036

Prostate Cancer:

Why It Is Different

Dr Peter Whelan

"If you have recently been diagnosed with prostate cancer, then you have still have plenty of time to make decisions."

Dr Peter Whelan

Prostate Cancer:

Why It Is Different

Dr Peter Whelan

Table of Contents

Preface

Introduction

1. What is the Prostate?

2. What is Prostate Cancer?

3. How Our Understanding of Prostate Cancer evolved: 1850 – 1980

4. Changes

5. The Rise

6. Consequences

7. Competition

8. A Re-examination of Hormones

9. New Techniques: I Robot

10. New Drugs

11. New Imaging

12. Active Surveillance, and the Search for Novel Therapies

13. What is to be Done?

Preface

Prostate cancer is not trivial and kills. In the last thirty years both the number of men diagnosed with the disease and of those whose deaths are attributed to it have steadily risen. Because all figures related to prostate cancer are contentious part of the impetus to write this book for the general public was to supply sufficient information so that anyone with the misfortune to receive a diagnosis of prostate cancer would be armed with the knowledge to be able to talk about their disease with their specialist and know that no harm was going to befall them, even if they took quite a considerable amount of time coming to a decision that was right for them, and probably for them only.

This is not like treating appendicitis. As will be shown as we move through this book, looking at what the prostate is, what it does and why it becomes diseased, we will see how prostate cancer has been treated in the past. How advances in understanding have shaped where we are now, and why 'what should I do?' is the most vital and important question that needs to be asked. Whether just dipping into parts of this book, or reading it straight through, it will become apparent just how difficult and complex a problem this presents, with the added burden that this cancer goes on for a couple of decades, at least. Individual weighing of odds and possibilities, knowing what goals an individual patient desires, and whether these are achievable are at the root of understanding, and the successful outcome of management. It will be noticed that the word 'cure' is not used, and this is deliberate.

When I began my surgical training, I was told that the art of the specialist was to ensure that your patient died of some other specialist's disease. In this age which eschews gallows' humour, the notion that I learnt later, and which still is applicable, was to make prostate cancer a chronic disease, which like heart diseases and diabetes could be controlled in many patients for a long time and that the patient could lead a normal life. I believe that this is still the ultimate goal.

There are no rogues or villains in this book. Some may have been a little 'fly' but always in the context of what was the general consensus, based on research evidence, of what was considered the best treatment, or possible treatments at a particular time. Retrospectively, there is always 20/20 vision.

In 1997 I published a paper in the *British Medical Journal* railing against the promiscuous use of the PSA blood test, as I saw it. This was decidedly not mainstream received wisdom at the time, but the journal published it in its best traditions of looking at all sides of an argument, and I continued to enjoy a richly rewarding career in urology, both nationally and internationally, being received with graciousness and courtesy by some of my colleagues whom I may criticise in this book and who certainly criticised me at the time.

Urologists are a special breed, I feel, and I have been proud to be one. Whether in Korea, Japan, America, Argentina, Europe, Russia, China, Egypt, anywhere, they have always appeared the same type of person, who care deeply for their patients but don't take themselves too seriously. As a former Deputy Governor of the Bank of England told us once as we were enlisting his help in fundraising, 'at bottom you'll always be plumbers.'

But this is a surgical specialty and many problems stem from 'car park credibility'. Are you not undertaking the surgery because you do not feel it appropriate in this patient or because you are frightened that you can't do the procedure? None of us is immune from these subliminal influences, although, fortunately, radical surgery for bladder cancer is recognised as a very big deal and I confess to buttressing my own credibility by doing many of these procedures. Similarly, I am not dismissive of 'heroic surgery' per se. Although the odds were that there was only a 0.6% chance of remission in a patient with kidney cancer which had spread everywhere, with so much disease in his lungs he needed oxygen, and the kidney cancer I removed was over 3 kgs, this 47 year-old, who was my age exactly at the time, was going nowhere. He survived, responded, and is still the same age as me more than 20 years later. I also remember, alas, the several similar patients who failed to respond, with the cancer taking its remorseless course, and most poignantly, a man with a large tumour and a debatable abnormality in his chest, who despite a successful operation was overwhelmed by his cancer, whatever my medical oncologist colleague and I did, never left hospital, and died four weeks after the operation; a major worry being whether the trauma of the surgery had actually precipitated its uncontrollable spread; he was only 53.

I have realised over the years the immense privilege it has been to work in the NHS in Great Britain. One of its founding principles, annunciated by Aneurin Bevan, its midwife, was that 'all professionals ...were to use your judgement and skills without hindrance...'For many reasons, which will be discussed, we have fallen away from that ideal, but in order that it may return, the patient needs to be as equal a partner in the discussions about what happens to them as possible. The hope is that this book will enable patients and potential patients to understand the process, understand the options, and to be enabled to make the best decision in their individual situation.

Introduction

No urologist doubts the efficacy and effectiveness of surgery in the management of urogenital cancer. At least 50% of patients with MIBC (muscle invasive bladder cancer) will be cured by radical surgery, in this case radical cystectomy, with most recurrences occurring within five years of initial treatment, and most urologists are happy to discharge patients as cured after ten years follow up, and some have argued for the safety of earlier discontinuation of review. Things are even better with renal (kidney) cancer in all its variants. Approximately 70% of patients are cured, most recurrences occur within two years and many patients can, with confidence, be discharged after five years of follow up. There are well-documented late recurrences, up to ten or more years after initial surgery, but these are rare, can frequently be treated by further surgery, and in no way justify all patients being followed up for many years, or indefinitely.

Even before 1978 when effective chemotherapy became available for testis cancer, a combination of surgery and radiation therapy had pushed the five-year survival from just over 50% in the 1950s to 67% by the late 1960s.

We know from wider studies in medicine that effective interventions cause a significant fall in death rates from disease, most notably what happened in cardiovascular disease where the death rate was halved.

We also know what an effective screening programme looks like when we note the fall in both the incidence and death rate in cervical cancer, the latter falling from 3,000 per year to 800 per year in the last twenty years or so.

Prostate cancer, the commonest malignancy in men, does not follow these easy paradigms, but presents us with a whole different order of difficulties, not least the paradox that men, as a group with the disease, live longer than those without. 'Get prostate cancer and live longer' is not the sort of slogan that is likely to either fill the coffers of prostate cancer-oriented charities or enable adequate funding to be obtained to investigate this disease and diminish the still significant death toll it imposes.

First, as we shall see, the diagnosis of prostate cancer in more than 90% of patients in the last couple of decades has been very early. Even a cursory glance at cancer information websites yields the facts that in low- and intermediate-risk patients, there appears to be a near 100% five- and ten-year survival. The ProTech study results of nearly 1,700 men randomly assigned to have surgery, radiation therapy or active surveillance yielded 4,5,and 8 deaths respectively at 10 years (1%) where many more patients had died of other causes, as one would expect in this group of men predominantly in the last quarter of their lives.

The 'gold standard' of therapeutic endeavour is the randomised controlled trial (RCT) of which there are precious few in prostate cancer. There are none in radiation therapy and its various offshoots such as brachytherapy, and more distantly focal therapy using various modalities, and only two in surgery: the US PIVOT trial which showed no difference between an actively treated surgical arm and active surveillance (there are many arguments about this study which will be looked at later, but the figures are true; the interpretation is in dispute), and the Scandinavian Trial, which at 20 years appeared to show an absolute benefit of about 11%, which meant that at least 7/8 patients did not derive any obvious benefit from their treatment. (Here again the results are arguable from many angles, but the systematic care with follow up of the investigators allows us to see the end-of-life outcome in the majority of these patients.)

What this short introductory review demonstrates beyond doubt is the very different way prostate cancer evolves from most cancers; that direct surgical intervention does not, as in other tumours, pay a fairly rapid dividend for the trauma and complications the treatment will inflict. Indeed, the complications are likely to be present for a very long time before the patient knows whether the sacrifice has been worth it. Only 10% of prostate cancers are diagnosed in men under 60, so that for most, actuarially, another disease is much more likely to prove fatal than prostate cancer. Are the side effects with a small chance of benefit fifteen or twenty years hence worth putting up with if they wreck a fit man's life for the next decade or more?

In the UK one of the most malevolent distractions from fully understanding how prostate cancer works has been the Cancer Plan, and its improving outcomes campaign, promulgated in 2002. Having struggled to understand and then articulate a set of standards for the three commonest cancers − breast, lung and colorectal − the authors of the plan shoehorned all other tumours into this template. The baleful effects of this lazy approach to all other cancers we still live with. However, the rest of the world has no such 'top down' diktat to hide behind, yet early diagnosis and treatment has until relatively recently been followed internationally.

It is the author's contention that failure to understand the natural history of prostate cancer has led to overdiagnosis and overtreatment, that the facts, such as they are, have been present for the better part of forty years, that many lives have been ruined by side effects of treatment with no compensating survival benefit and that a much more nuanced approach is vital if another generation of fit men in their 60s and 70s are not to suffer the same fate.

This is a disease of the last quarter of a man's life; of the 10,000 or so deaths attributed to prostate cancer in the UK per annum, only 15 cases were reported in the 40-49-year-old bracket, and only about 650 in the cohort 50 -59. These are young men with thirty or forty years ahead of them; a predictable cure should add to and enhance their lives. Within the UK (and the figures are similar elsewhere in Europe and North America) men have begun to get sick and are already on multiple medications, over four different drugs in nearly half of cases, once they get into their 60s. Given the length the disease will have to run in the majority of men, and that competing mortalities will trump death from prostate cancer, it is, I believe, essential that men and their relatives understand very clearly what they are signing up for, whichever one of the bewildering range of options they choose or are encouraged to take.

In a very large important study of patient-reported outcomes (PROMS) most patients who had active treatment, whatever the modality − surgery, radiation therapy or other − reported a great many side effects and were not surprisingly depressed. At two years, whilst many of the side effects persisted the patients reported themselves much happier despite ongoing problems. Two possibilities exist to explain this outcome. Their lives have been saved and they would have died without treatment, although there is absolutely no evidence anywhere to support that contention with prostate cancer; the other is that they thought they would die without treatment and no one offered an alternative viewpoint.

Finding themselves alive two years down the line would make anyone happy.

New diagnostic technologies now in place will help, and new approaches to therapy will target those who could benefit, but it is necessary to understand how we got to where we are now, how some steps could have been avoided, and why only an individualised approach in this particular cancer can hope to serve each patient to enable them to have as trouble-free a life as possible, eschewing both the physical and psychological side effects by treating each patient's needs and concerns on their individual merits.

Let us first consider what the prostate is and what it does, briefly how it changes as men age, and then go on to consider how prostate cancer was treated in the past to allow us to understand how the present recommendations for treatment came about.

1. What is the Prostate?

The word prostate is a construct from two Greek words meaning 'one who stands before', neatly capturing the place of the prostate standing before the male bladder. When not diseased the prostate is about the size of a chestnut or apricot and weighs between 20 and 30 grams. It develops from the urogenital sinus and acquires glandular epithelia, connective tissue and smooth muscle cells by differentiation, such that by 9 weeks *in utero* it is plainly visible as a gland. It grows as the boy gets older but receives its accelerated push at puberty under the testosterone surge. Changes in the prostate thereafter, and most often dictated by disease, will be reviewed in the more general discussion of prostate cancer in the next chapter.

The anatomical description of the prostate has undergone several changes over the last seventy or so years, not only to try to better understand its function but also to more fully appreciate its situation in relation to adjoining structures such as the bladder and rectum, as well as the more closely associated structures such as the seminal vesicles, and how effective treatment may be applied to the diseased prostate.

The Barcelona surgeon Salvador Gil-Vernet was first to describe the close approximation of the nerves and blood vessels to the periphery of the prostate (1964), which not only served to supply and stimulate the prostate but were responsible for the control of both continence and erectile function. It was, however, Walsh and Donker (1982) who first demonstrated an anatomical approach to performing radical surgery, which Patrick Walsh carried out at Johns Hopkins Hospital in Baltimore in March 1982.

Similarly, Gil-Vernet (1953) laid the groundwork for the different zones of the prostate which was elaborated by John McNeal of San Francisco into the zones of the prostate which are recognised and utilised now. These are:

The Transitional Zone − is in the middle of the gland and makes up the smallest of the zones, being about 10% of total prostatic volume. It surrounds the urethra between the bladder and the upper third of the urethra. It is here that BPH develops and where only a small percentage of cancers are found.

The Central Zone – This surrounds the transitional zone and makes up to 20-25% of the prostate volume. This is where the duct, common to the prostate, seminal vesicle and seminal ducts, known as the ejaculatory duct, is found.

The Peripheral Zone – represents the major mass of the prostate, surrounds the other two zones and where the majority of prostate cancers are located.

The Anterior Fibro Muscular Zone – This is found just behind the pubic bone and makes up 5% or less of the total prostate volume. Few, if any, cancers are reported found here.

The descriptions of the ducts into which smaller ducts from the prostate gland cells secrete fluid exemplify the primary function of the prostate gland. The ducts enter into the prostatic urethra just before the external sphincter, which is part of the pelvic floor and consists of striated muscle, the same that is used to move our limbs and head. The internal sphincter is at the bladder neck and is made of smooth muscle. When ejaculation occurs, the internal sphincter automatically closes, whilst the external one opens to allow semen to exit. When the man passes urine, both sphincters open to allow the bladder to be evacuated.

The first function of the prostate is to contribute fluid to ejaculate. It is estimated that the prostatic contribution comprises 30-35% of ejaculated volume. It is alkaline and contributes to the chances of the sperm surviving in the acidic environment of the vagina.

Allied to this, the enzyme PSA (Prostate Specific Antigen), which is secreted by the lining (or luminal) cells of the prostatic ducts, enables sperm to swim by keeping the seminal fluid liquid and counteracting the 'clotting' tendency of fluid from the seminal vesicle. The muscle fibres within the prostate gland also enable the pumping action of the ejaculatory prostate to project its fluid a considerable distance, thus also contributing to maximising the chances of fertilisation. The effect of these contractions is to produce sexual satisfaction.

Vigorous massage of the prostate can produce the same effect of both ejaculation and sexual satisfaction, and in the past was the mainstay of treating chronic inflammations of the prostate. It is quite possible to gain significant control of this muscular action, as indeed, with any muscular activity, and in both Taoist and Tantric advanced practices, a dry ejaculate may be achieved by selectively closing the external sphincter which is under striated, or voluntary muscle control, which automatically by reflex then opens the internal sphincter and allows the sperm to go back into the bladder. We will examine this in a little more detail when we look at the normal mechanisms of micturition and ejaculation that the prostate participates in.

The name of prostate, indicating one who stands before, indicates its important but as yet incompletely understood role, firstly filtering toxins which may be in the sperm, and secondly stopping ascending infections from the urethra.

Within and closely adherent to the prostate are the nerves that not only innervate the prostate and facilitate its functions but also the nerves that enable erections to occur. This important phenomenon will be discussed several times in the context of how prostate cancer is treated.

The role of the prostate in reducing urinary tract infections (UTIs) is difficult to assess. The length of the male urethra and the effects of the urinary stream 'hosing out' bacteria has traditionally been the explanation of why men do not often get UTIs, and why men who develop bladder outflow obstruction with its consequent poor flow do become subject to them, but as we will increasingly discover with the prostate and all its works, a lineal relationship of cause and effect is rarely ever true.

The final role, and from the perspective of a healthy prostate and what happens to it when it becomes cancerous, is its role in the action and production of the male hormone testosterone. Testosterone produced by the testes is absorbed into the cells of the prostate where it is broken down to dihydrotestosterone by the action of the enzyme 5 alpha reductase, which has a tenfold greater activity than testosterone itself. It is necessary to keep prostate tissue healthy and active.

The prostate is subject to three main types of disease: infections and inflammations, benign prostatic hypertrophy or hyperplasia, and prostate cancer. All may coexist so that symptoms attributed to one or other of these two images are rarely of diagnostic significance or help.

Infections of the prostate are most commonly thought to be due to ascending infections, and with the prostatitis that affects young men, this is usually a sexually transmitted disease in which chlamydia and gonorrhoea are the most common. There was a small spike of bacterial infections, often associated with urinary tract infections, which was ascribed to the greater practice of anal intercourse, due to direct ascending infection from bowel organisms, and occasionally systemic bacterial infections such as staphylococcus aureus have given rise to prostatic infections and even abscesses. The prostate appears to act as a reservoir or safe place for infections as they may persist in the prostate for many years. A great deal of research and innumerable hypotheses about why the prostate accommodates these foreign bodies have been produced, to date without a definitive explanation. Of relevance to the way a cancer works the ability of foreign bodies of inflammation to sit symbiotically within the prostate, not be recognised by the body's immune system and so excite some form of inflammatory reaction, has been known for nearly fifty years, yet why it happens, and what, if anything, it means, remains elusive.

Benign prostatic hypertrophy (BPH) develops in the transitional zone of the prostate. It is under some degree of hormone control, and indeed one of the active drug therapies for this is a 5 alpha reductase inhibitor which shrinks the prostate gland over some months, but only by a fairly predictable percentage, approximately 40%,which is frequently therapeutically helpful but does not reduce this to a residual entity. BPH can grow to quite large proportions; glands of over 200g in size from a baseline of 20-30 have frequently been described, but the important point is that the peripheral zone of the gland is squeezed so that enucleation of the gland, by whatever means, the physical removal of the gland, remains the goal of interventional therapy if drug treatment fails. The area with the highest chances of harbouring a prostate cancer remains, and the risk remains undiminished.

The prostate participates in two important, indeed vital, activities in men; micturition and ejaculation. Micturition is initiated by a bladder reflex that if left unopposed will start a bladder contraction which aims to empty the bladder. To facilitate this action both the internal sphincter at the bladder neck and the external sphincter, which is just beyond the verumontanum, where the ejaculatory duct enters the urethra, are reflexly opened. The external sphincter can override this reflex at any time, the toilets burning down for example, but one of the signature symptoms of BPH is that the urine trapped between the internal and external sphincters, which when we are younger is pushed back into the bladder, is trapped for a short period and then the external sphincter opens to release this small amount of urine. Hence, the common symptom amongst older men of 'post-micturition dribbling' which is characterised by a gap in flow before further urine; usually only a small amount is released suddenly and uncontrollably.

If the prostate is removed completely or rendered inoperative in its functions, then the consequences are predictable. The therapy of prostate cancer has been a constant conflict between eliminating a cancer which could prove fatal and the consequences to the man of problems of micturition control and preserving sexual function. How this conflict has played out in the past, and continues to play out contemporaneously, is the subject of this book.

2. What is Prostate Cancer?

The popular image of what constitutes a cancer is a mixture of a vague knowledge of lung and breast cancer. Lung cancer appears the archetypal form of cancer, diagnosed late, remorselessly progressive, affected little by any form of therapy, and often running a relatively short course to its inevitable, fatal outcome. Statistics would support this contention. In 2016 there were 46,388 new cases registered of lung cancer and 35,620,deaths reported from lung cancer; at 10 years post- diagnosis barely 5 % of patients were still alive, and as can be seen from the statistics survival for many patients with this cancer is measured in months, or a year or so, at best.

Breast cancer shows another side to contemporary views of what cancer is. It, as well as being the commonest cancer to affect women (55,122 new cases diagnosed in 2016 with 11,563 deaths from the disease in the same year), appears to have been much better managed, as 78% of patients are alive at 10 years. Many notable women from numerous walks of life have fallen victim to the disease, have charted and recorded their individual experiences, and with its high media profile news about breast cancer is rarely out of sight. It also seems to confirm many people's feelings about cancer. Getting it early ensures a better chance of cure, although there remains a vigorous debate about whether breast screening has helped or harmed more women (Cochrane Collaborative, 2013) and the results currently still remain equivocal; new treatments, especially the use of hormones have made a considerable difference to outcomes; new modes of surgery, including reconstructive surgery, have enabled treatments to be better accepted and focused on cure, and rehabilitation with dignity.

When one moves to consider prostate cancer, it is not surprising that one or two of these images come to mind. In 2016 47,151 cases were registered, with 11,631 deaths ascribed to it. At 10 years 84% of patients were alive, better by a small amount than breast cancer, significantly better than the 57% for bowel cancer, the fourth most numerous cancer, and a world away from the dire outlook for lung cancer. With a little additional knowledge one hears that there is a blood test to assist early diagnosis, active intervention by surgery or radiation therapy is available, and that this situation has been in place for nearly twenty years; there would seem very little that need alarm us in the current management of the disease, and the sure expectation that the impressive figure of 84% will gradually increase as new therapies are introduced. It is impressive for a male cancer, given that it usually takes a coach and horses to get males to see a doctor. The system, or rather systems worldwide, as they are replicated and sometimes even better, in other high-income countries, is also impressive.

So why the problem, and a book like this? Like so many things in life nothing is as it first appears and in the case of prostate cancer this is true in a whole lot of unexpected ways.

To start at the beginning, is prostate cancer common? The recorded incidence has steadily risen over the last forty years worldwide. In 1980 there were approximately 17,500 new diagnoses in the UK, and 8,000 deaths. In the USA the comparable figures were 101,000 new cases and approximately 30,000 deaths. At the beginning of the 1990s more aggressive screening using the blood test Prostate Specific Antigen (PSA) led to a spike in incidence with approaching 400,000 cases diagnosed in US in one year, but since then the rate has fallen back to its new baseline of 240,000 cases a year or so. In 1992 the US had recorded 132,000 new cases, with 34,000 deaths. The UK followed American practice in both diagnostics and treatments, but these were introduced somewhat later and there is a lag period before UK statistics mirror those of the USA. Despite the two and a half times more cases now being diagnosed there were still 29,554 deaths due to prostate cancer in 2003 and the projected number of deaths for 2018 is 29,430.

These figures are obviously open to a great many different interpretations. Despite the increased number of cases being found no more are dying than 40 years ago and presumably many more are being cured than previously. Despite earlier diagnosis (over 90% are early, confined tumours) we are not getting the appropriate treatment to the most at risk men, or all our early detection has managed to achieve is to find tumours that might have done all right if left alone, so that in spite of the large numbers of cancers treated we are still struggling to deliver the appropriate treatment for each individual tumour. When active intervention works, as with cardio-vascular disease, the mortality from that entity is halved (Peeters 2012). However we dress it up, the same actual number of men are dying from prostate cancer, and as we can see from the UK results, more are dying now from prostate cancer than forty years ago. Why?

Before diving into statistics, efficacies of health care systems, the neglect of men, and any number of emotive topics, we will start by considering the nature and natural history of prostate cancer.

The Nature of Prostate Cancer

The epithelial or lining cells of the prostatic ductules and ducts give rise to 90% of prostate cancer, and it is these tumours that exhibit the characteristics which we will mainly discuss further. Other pathological types arising from this tissue include arcomatoid and small cell lesions, as well as urothelial cancers arising from the lining of the urethra passing through the prostate. The non-epithelial and stromal elements produce their own type of tumour, such as leiomyosarcomas and solitary fibrous tumours, but these are all uncommon and frequently require a different approach to therapy. The aim of this book is to examine the common prostate cancer, and hereafter, that is all we will be discussing.

Natural History of Prostate Cancer

Prostate cancer is predominantly a disease of older men. Isolated cases only have been reported in the third and fourth decades, and even in men's forties the numbers in the UK, for example, are rarely above 20. When, however, does the cancer become initiated and can we gain any clue as to how long it takes for a prostate malignancy to become clinically active? The natural history of any cancer is observation of its growth without intervention. Knowledge of this allows the treating clinician to offer a prognosis, and to indicate where each therapy will impact, and how effectively, and for how long that impact will last.

The first indication that prostate cancer might possess unique features came in an autopsy study by Moore (1935), who found in a range of elderly men who had died from non-malignant causes 17% had identifiable areas of prostate cancer which had not contributed at all to the death of the patient and, indeed, appeared to be lying indolently in the prostate. Much greater notice was taken of a similar finding reported in 1954 by Franks. This was because the figure he reported was 38% and in albeit a relatively small group of autopsies apparently established what had been clinically known, that prostate cancer was associated with increasing age, and the older one became the more likely it was that these lesions were to be found in the prostate. From their appearance alone, it was not possible to distinguish a clinically active but well-differentiated tumour from one sitting contentedly in the prostate and apparently harming no one. Only when the cells of the tumour became recognisably more disorganised and began flooding across tissue planes were these always seen as clinically significant.

The phenomenon, of a large volume of possible tumour, with only a small amount, like an iceberg, showing above the waterline, or clinically active, meant that searching out these lesions was not a priority; especially when compared to any other tumour, there was effective treatment for widespread or metastatic cancer, and given the sometimes brutal reality of contemporary treatment for local disease, not one that either patient or physician actively sought. An interesting glimpse of what might be going on was furnished by Sadr (1994) who reviewed the histology of just under 200 prostates from autopsy specimens in young men who had died violently, from road traffic accidents, suicides and criminal assault. He felt that he was able to identify the presence of prostatic interepithelial neoplasia (PIN) of high grade in a significant minority of these men who were all under forty. Surprisingly, the incidence appeared to be the same for blacks and whites. It remains a matter of continuing debate as to whether this entity is a genuine premalignant condition and also demonstrates how difficult such painstaking work is and how hard it would be to recruit meaningful numbers.

In 1969 Barnes found a series of 86 men who had been diagnosed with confined prostate cancer at his institution between 1930 and 1961 and had received no active therapy. In this retrospective study he found that 50% were still alive at 10 years from diagnosis and 30% alive at 15 years. He noted, most importantly, in this group that at least two thirds had died of conditions other than prostate cancer. Given the small sample and the retrospective analysis large claims would be difficult to justify, but he did express the opinion that these results with current clinical observations suggested that active treatment, i.e. surgery or radiation therapy was probably unhelpful and probably deleterious to patients with a life expectancy of less than ten years.

In 1994 Chodak and colleagues reported on the conservative management of 828 patients collected from a number of centres and subjected to a pooled analysis. In this they measured the disease- specific survival (how many did not die from prostate cancer) at 10 years, not the overall survival. They showed that 87% in low grade and 34% in high grade met their outcome criteria. During this period of observation 81% low grade cancers at diagnosis remained metastases free, whereas only 26% of those with high grade disease were metastases free. This raised the spectre of what will become increasingly familiar to us as the paradox that in the good risk group, while most conformed to prediction, about 20%, despite the initial favourable circumstance did go on to progress and be life threatening, whilst the high-risk group also conformed to expectations but with a significant minority, a quarter, failing to progress. What this observational study did reemphasise was that even with high-risk disease there is time to think about what to do.

In 1997 Johansson reported a prospective cohort study of 223 Swedish men diagnosed with localised prostate cancer, in whom any initial treatment was deferred. This group was assiduously followed for over three decades (Johansson [2004], Popiolek [2013]). It was found that all these patients had good disease-specific survival up to 15 years, 76.9% had survived without evidence of metastases, but in the next five years, the disease-specific survival declined to 54.4%. As per the stated protocol patients who progressed were treated with hormones and no treatment was given to patients who remained stable. In 2011, when the study had lasted 32 years and only three of the original patients survived, a further, final analysis of the data was undertaken. 142 men of the 223 (64%) remained untreated for their prostate cancer before dying of other causes. In contrast to this good, majority group, 38/79 men treated with hormones died of prostate cancer, and it is their group who managed to skew the figures at 20 years. After 20 years with the numbers of survivors diminishing there was no further increase in progression. In summary, most patients needed no treatment for their prostate cancer, and even in the third that progressed and were treated with hormones (as we will see, a purely palliative therapy), half did not die from prostate cancer. This study was important, and probably unrepeatable because the schedule was set out prospectively and the protocol adhered to. It is therefore probably one of the few reflections of the natural history of the disease, and again re-emphasises its longevity. In 2005 Albertsen reported on a retrospective study of 767 patients followed for a mean of 24 years with watchful waiting; this showed at 15 years no significant difference in the rate of progression or mortality, but the grade of tumour, how aggressive it was, made a decided difference. They used a measure of deaths per 1,000 patient years. In the high-risk group the deaths were 121 per 1,000 patient years, whilst in the low-risk group it was 6 deaths per 1,000 patient years.

This review of the natural history brings several factors into clarity. Prostate cancer is a long slow disease, as compared with many cancers, making statements about cure difficult over short time scales. A lot of disease shows no clinical symptoms, and most patients succumb from some other disease process long before their prostate cancer. However, this is a cancer and patients perceived to have high-risk disease do suc-cumb to prostate cancer, but even here no nice clear separation is pos-sible; an individual is a 100% and has only one run at this, but the fact that good may occasionally go bad, and bad is not always fatal merely displays the depths of our ignorance.

Other factors are known to have a bearing on the chances of devel-oping prostate cancer, but all contribute rather than being pivotal, as far as we know, to this change.

Old Age

Prostate cancer has always been known as the cancer of old age. Prior to the PSA era (to be discussed in greater detail later, but taken as from 1990 onwards), in 1980 70% were diagnosed over the age of 70 in Den-mark, with the results similar in most high-income countries, which with the use of PSA has changed thirty years later to only 49% being over 70 at diagnosis, still making it, however, predominantly a disease of the last quarter of life. What is not found anywhere is a cohort of young men, un-der forty for example, as you can get with women for breast cancer, and until men are into their fifties the numbers of cases anywhere are in the few dozens or scores at worst.

Family /Hereditary Associations

A strong correlation with increased risk of prostate cancer and relatives such as fathers and brothers having the disease has been identified for some time (Whittemore 1995) and increasing work has been done with families with numbers of cases to elucidate risk and to study possible ge-netic patterns, such as the large group of UK cases investigated by Ros Eeles at the Royal Marsden Hospital. Recently Blatt (2016) has reviewed the very comprehensive available Swedish data and has produced some absolute risk values together in the paper from Sweden with some picto-graphs giving a visual display about what sort of risk there is. They showed if there was both a father and brother with prostate cancer, then the risk was twice that for a remaining male and a 30% chance of the dia-gnosis before 75 compared with a 13% chance of the latter in a man with no family history. There also appeared to be a 9% risk of getting an ag-gressive tumour compared to the general population of 5%. It is the heightened risk overall and the chance of an unfavourable outcome that leads to most being recommended to seek further investigation. Things are sometimes difficult.

Patient A was a recently retired doctor whose elder brother had died from prostate cancer and after further research into the family history it was found that both his father and uncle had been diagnosed with pro-state cancer, although the father had apparently died of heart disease. Patient A sought advice and had a PSA (Prostate Specific Antigen blood test; a great deal more about this in due course) which came back at 0.2 (range 0-4 or 0-3; more about this too). His GP examined him and felt his prostate gland was normal. Unhappy with this, he gained a special-ist's opinion. He agreed that per rectal examination the prostate felt nor-mal and recommended against any further action other than a repeat PSA in six months. He explained that biopsying the prostate was not a benign process with up to 4% of patients in some series being admitted with sepsis, and there could be up to one in ten deaths from septicaemia. Patient A nevertheless pursued matters further until he found a radiolo-gist who would carry out the biopsies with patient A writing a waiver clause should any complications ensue. None did, and the six core biopsies all showed high grade prostate cancer (Gleason 8, again to be explained in due time). Strangely patient A then found it difficult to get his preferred treatment, radical surgery, being steered towards radiation therapy, because cases with high risk disease tended to do less well. Pa-tient A eventually found a younger urologist who also believed that if surgery was any good it must help those with high-risk disease. Fortu-nately, patient A's prostate's margins were clear of tumour. There en-sued one final, earnest discussion. The usual follow up was with PSA blood tests. Patient A felt these would be a waste of time as the PSA had been unmeasurable virtually at the beginning of these events. He negoti-ated a follow-up process that consisted of annual bone scans, or sooner if he felt symptoms, as 90% of metastases went to bone and refused any additional therapy. He, I believe, remains fit and well.

I would like you to keep this case in mind as we review the history of our understanding of prostate cancer, and we discuss contemporary treatments so that we are able to explore why he had such a problem, all opinions he received being justified by some part of the accumulated literature.

In passing, it is worth noting that this case spread by the rumour mill, so unusual was it, but that is frequently the way medicine has staggered forward by means of unusual case reports; in the current age of impact factors many medical journals have dropped their case reports but some still retain them, thank goodness, and Ian Pearce, the editor of the UK Journal of Clinical Urology, devoted a whole issue to these types of cases. On the day a British urologist had removed the wrong kidney and his case was subsequently all over the national press, sitting on my ward waiting to have her left kidney tumour removed was a lady with *citus inversus*. This is a rare condition in which the heart is on the right side not the left, the liver on the left and not the right and so forth. This lady's peculiar twist was to have her heart in the correct position on the left but underneath the diaphragm; the organs were reversed. You may imagine there was a decided slowness, even with all the imaging, before the correct kidney with its tumour in it was removed.

Race and Ethnicity

Race appears a significant risk factor with regard to both incidence of disease and mortality from it. It has been known for some time that black Americans had a higher incidence than white and also an increased mortality from the disease. Formerly this was considered to be due to both poor socio-economic conditions for the blacks compared with the white population on average, but also to a possible higher incidence of chronic prostatic infections, although elements of this seemed to be due to caricature and lazy racism. However, even when these factors are controlled, black Americans are 1.6 times more likely to develop prostate cancer, and twice as likely to die from prostate cancer as whites (SEER data 2000-2006). A further study (Albain 2009) also tried to control for socio-economic factors by examining the outcomes of prostate cancer patients who had participated in a variety of trials by the Southwest Oncology Group (SWOG) and found that blacks had a 21% greater chance of dying than whites in the same protocol. Much more research is obviously needed.

In contrast Americans of Asian origin appear to have a lesser susceptibility to prostate cancer. From the same SEER data their rate was just over half that of whites, and their mortality from the disease was five times less likely than American blacks. Hispanics have a rate slightly lower than whites but is broadly similar for incidence and mortality. Some of this difference could be related to diet.

Diet

Earlier studies had shown a low incidence of prostate cancer in both Chinese and Japanese and was thought to be possibly related to the predominant diet in these countries. A meta-analysis of several case control studies and two cohort studies suggested that soy reduced the risk of prostate cancer in males with a high soy consumption and might explain the lower incidence in Asian males; especially when a small study appeared to suggest that in ethnic Japanese who had moved to California or been born there, the risk of prostate cancer rose towards the expected white population rate (Yan.2005). In a study in 2014 a California-based group looked at six different Asian racial groups: Chinese American-born and overseas-born, Japanese in the same two categories, and overseas-born Filipinos and Vietnamese. Surprisingly, their figures suggested there was now an increased risk of prostate cancer compared to whites across all groups, small in the Japanese, but approaching the risk of American blacks for Filipinos. All these studies, as their authors readily admit, are susceptible to selection bias. Lycopenes, which are an active ingredient of tomatoes, were thought to have a role in reducing prostate cancer risk in people eating Mediterranean diets. Sadly, a case-control study (Peters,2007) did not find any such reduction.

One of the longest running studies as to whether dietary supplements (these were selenium and vitamin E {SELECT trial})would be beneficial, appeared initially promising, but an update in 2014 (Thompson) found that selenium had no effect on prostate cancer occurrence whilst vitamin E had a detrimental effect, as it produced more cancers than the control arm. This trial had run for nearly two decades and re-emphasises again that answers are a long time coming, and initial benefits may be erroneous.

Chronic Infection

Most prostate glands when examined have areas of chronic inflammation but whether these contribute to formation of prostate cancer remains an active area of research. Many men are treated for clinical prostatitis when young, and some may require frequent treatment for the symptoms of chronic prostatitis over many years, but no one so far has shown a lineal relationship to this problem and the development of prostate cancer. We know some cancers develop after the constant irritation which inflammation, for example, could supply, and there could be many subclinical cases of inflammation, but tumours derived from chronic inflammation tend to be squamous carcinomas, not adenocarcinomas we find in the prostate.

Hormones

A great deal of research has dealt with the need for the prostate to have the presence of androgens in order to grow and function. The pivotal work of Charles Huggins in this respect, which won him the Nobel prize for medicine, will be reviewed in detail in due course, but confirmation of this was provided by Jie Ping Wu, a pupil of Huggins in Chicago in the 1930s who set up the first dedicated urology unit in Beijing. In 1960 there were still 26 eunuchs in Beijing surviving from the Qing dynasty which had been overthrown in 1912. This group of men, who had been castrated between the ages of 10 and 26, were now mostly in their seventies and old. Wu showed that clinically the prostate was impalpable in all, and none had developed prostate cancer. However, perfect symmetry, as ever in medicine, was not achieved. In 1991 Boccon-Gibod, in Paris, described the presence of prostate cancer in a man who had undergone chemical castration thirty-five years previously voluntarily after conviction for sexual offences, a common offering to such prisoners in Europe and North America in the first half of the twentieth century, and a more instructive case report from 2016 (Stocking) reported the case of a man who had suffered mumps orchitis at the age of 13. He had developed secondary sex characteristics, but late, and had had an unsatisfactory marriage. He was treated for hypertension in his fifties and at age 60 was recommended to go on to testosterone supplements with his pre-treatment PSA being 0.2. When the PSA some while later was 0.43 he had an ultrasound scan of his prostate, which suggested a cancer, and subsequent biopsies confirmed a high-risk Gleason 8 tumour. He subsequently underwent a radical prostatectomy. The implications of this case, and the practice reported, will be discussed when we look at contemporary therapies.

If, sixty years ago, a discussion took place about what influences the possibility of prostate cancer, it would be no different from today's discussion. It is a disease of the aging male; then most cases were diagnosed after the age of 70. Black Americans were at higher risk although the reasons conjectured but not proven; and there might be something in both different racial origins, an apparent lower risk in Asian males, but this might also be linked to a vegetarian diet but again the protective elements were unknown. At this time, sixty years ago, there was a proven and consistent palliative treatment, the reduction of male hormones which was unique to metastatic, or widespread cancer. This palliative treatment lasted for a couple of years at worst, and many years at best. Given the multiple, competing morbidities leading to mortalities in this age group, consensus opinion felt this cancer could at least be parked, and efforts to treat and hopefully cure be directed at tumours affecting young people, and those in middle age, whose lives were being cut short, and in whom most remedies simply did not work.

Although from a public health perspective, castration of all males over forty might have prevented most cases of prostate cancer, a very decided consensus among experts, all of whom were men, concluded this was far too drastic a move to even discuss, given the cancer's known characteristics, and the fact that it was a minority that had the misfortune to suffer the disease. Prevention, or possibly cure, under any circumstances was not just a bridge but a whole ocean too far.

3. How Our Understanding of Prostate Cancer Evolved: 1850-1980

Most surgical histories, especially British ones, always start with one of the innumerable observations of John Hunter; prostate cancer is no exception. In 1786 he recorded his observations on the seasonal change in size of the prostate and testes of several dogs, the shrinkage effects of castration, and felt that there was solid enough evidence to link the testes and the development of secondary sexual characteristics. It was, however, J Adam, a surgeon at the London Hospital in Whitechapel, who in a case report published in the *Lancet*, initiated formal treatment of a cancerous prostate. He describes a case 'of scirrhous of the prostate gland with accompanying affliction of the lymphatic glands in the lumbar region and the pelvis'. He had difficulty in forging a passageway through the very hard tissue into the bladder and suggests that this is a quite rare manifestation of prostatic disease.

In 1869 Buchler described a smaller circumscribed tumour of the prostate for which he had performed a partial prostatectomy via the perineum (the area between the scrotum and the anus, the historical route for urological surgeons cutting for the stone, from ancient times, through Frere Jacques and John Cheselden, to Thompson who had operated on Napoleon III). In 1883 Leisrink carried out the complete removal of the prostate via the perineal route and re-anastomosed or joined the urethra at the external sphincter to the bladder neck. In 1904 Hugh Hampton Young, of Johns Hopkins, defined the anatomy of this procedure more clearly showing the importance of making the join of the urethra and bladder neck needed to be above the sphincter (supra-sphincteric) to ensure a reasonable chance of continence. With some additional modifications by Belt, amongst others, this remained the standard operation for localised prostate cancer for 40 years. In the best hands there was a 30% incidence of urinary incontinence and 100% of the men were impotent postoperatively.

The transvesical route used for BPH was tried for clinically cancerous lesions, but there was no separation of planes and incontinence was very frequent, and it was soon discarded. In 1945 the British surgeon Terence Millin demonstrated the retropubic approach for both the treatment of BPH, in which the capsule of the prostate was opened and the enlarged prostate enucleated, and for removal of a cancerous prostate, whereby the prostate was operated upon outside the prostate and the gland removed totally. The operative complications were broadly similar to the perineal operation but became more popular in view of the surgeon's greater experience with this approach because of the large number of benign cases that were treated. Here the situation remained for the next thirty years or so.

Radiation therapy to treat localised prostate cancer was a little slower in being adopted, mainly for technical reasons. In 1904 a case report from France showed the first successful use of x-ray therapy to treat a locally advanced prostate cancer. In 1908, again from France, a report showed that a catheter with radium seed within it could be positioned in the prostatic urethra and radiation delivered to the tumour. Length of exposure was purely arbitrary. In 1923 'deep' x-rays were used to treat the pain from bony metastases of prostate cancer with some success in pain control.

The problem with all these early attempts was that the x-rays used relied on low energy beams, which meant that they lacked depth of penetration, and therefore gave rise to severe skin burns, in some of which radiation-induced skin cancers arose. Usage was, not unexpectedly, very low in the first half of the twentieth century.

Important discoveries in radiation science led to new developments in radiotherapy. Following the promulgation of the subatomic particle acceleration theory and the creation of particle accelerators called 'linacs', these new machines were found to produce megavoltage x-rays that offered deeper skin penetration, and importantly, a skin-sparing effect. This allowed higher doses of radiation to be delivered without the previously seen skin toxicity. In 1953 an 8-megavoltage (MV) linac was installed at the Hammersmith Hospital, London, which began to treat various tumours, of which prostate cancer was one. The era of external beam radiotherapy (EBRT) had arrived. During the 1950s and beyond, Malcolm Bagshaw from Stanford in the USA, refined therapy for prostate cancer specifically and achieved some notable results. Again, there was a period of stability with this use of 2D (dimensional) radiotherapy being standard before the next technological breakthrough.

Meanwhile the possible interplay between the hormones affecting the prostate, principally testosterone, and the prostate was further elaborated. In 1893 White, a surgeon from Philadelphia, advocated the use of castration for the treatment of obstructed bladders. This met with variable clinical success with regards to the shrinkage of the prostate achieved and hence the chances of the obstruction being relieved, but it did not find a ready receptive patient base.

In the early part of the twentieth century animal experiments showed the relationship between the pituitary gland, just beneath the brain, the testes and the prostate. A. Gutman was one of several scientists who showed the action of phosphatase, and that there were at least two types, acid functioning at a ph of 4.6 and alkaline, functioning at a ph of 9.3. This enabled further work by Alexander and Ethel Gutman in the early 1930s to show that acid phosphatase was consistently elevated in men who demonstrated bone metastases from prostate cancer, and that the alkaline phosphatase was also frequently elevated. In 1935 Deming showed that normal prostate tissue became atrophic in primates after castration whereas BPH was unaffected. In 1938 Moore and McLellen showed the same effects when oestrogens were used. These findings set the stage for the seminal discoveries of Charles Huggins in two papers in 1941.

The generally accepted concept concerning cancer growth was that the cells had become autonomous and became wilder in shape, size and number as the tumour grew. Only radiation ablation, or surgical removal, was effective in altering the progress of the tumour. What Huggins was able to demonstrate was that even though prostate cancer cells exhibited all these traits, the tumour was still under hormonal control. In classical experiments he showed that the prostate tumours shrank on withdrawal of androgens, and to complete the cycle showed that castration or orchidectomy, and oestrogen drugs were equivalent. He further showed that acid phosphatase acted as a marker, falling as the cancer diminished, and rising again once the effects of the hormones or castration waned. He treated 21 patients with prostate cancer, 8 of whom had metastases; all responded, and 4 of the patients with localised disease lived for more than 12 years. He noted in the bone metastatic group that alkaline phosphatase remained elevated for some time after responding and appeared to reflect bone healing as the presence of metastases became hard to see on x-rays as the level fell.

Huggins received the Nobel Prize for Medicine in 1966. In essence the whole way prostate cancer was managed flowed from these observations, which were replicated over and over again. As well as defining how the patient could be treated, and that responses occurred even in the most advanced cases, he also cautioned that some time along the course of the tumour's history it began to overcome the effects of androgen withdrawal and that further treatments would be necessary.

It is difficult to convey the almost magical effect this treatment had, especially on patients with very large burdens of metastatic cancer, affecting all their bones and making them anaemic. Within days, they literally 'took up their beds and walked'. Because this had been developed by a urologist, and because the treatments of prostate cancer — surgery, orchidectomy, oestrogen medication — could be given, and were all given by urologists, patients with prostate cancer tended in most countries to stay with their urologist just as heart or diabetic patients remained with their specialists. If patients opted for radiotherapy, this was a one-off therapy, and if supplemental treatment became necessary, because the treatment had failed, they came back under the care of the urologist, for palliative care. Interestingly, it was only at the beginning of the twenty-first century that medical oncologists became involved in the care of this particular group of cancer patients.

Huggins, in the early 1950s, devoted his research efforts to breast cancer, which he felt had similar hormonal controls. The systematic use of tamoxifen in breast cancer patients in the 1990s eventually gave women sufferers the hormone boost in therapeutic terms that men with prostate cancer had enjoyed for almost fifty years.

Over the next thirty years the practical management of prostate cancer altered little. At least half the patients presented with advanced disease and were treated with some form of androgen deprivation therapy (ADT) whilst the others presented incidentally, cancer being found in their prostates which had been removed for urinary symptoms and presumed to have been caused by BPH, or just occasionally a chance rectal examination revealed a suspicious prostate which proved to be cancerous on biopsy.

In 1960 Byar, the statistician for the Veterans' Administration Co-operative Urological Research Group (VACURG), designed a series of randomised, prospective, controlled trials to identify the optimal treatment of prostate cancer with hormones. The first study examined DES (diethylstilboestrol) at 5mgs and 1mg, versus orchiectomy plus placebo, and orchidectomy plus DES, versus placebo. The second looked more carefully at 1 mg DES and the last compared DES with Premarin (conjugated equine oestrogen) and Provera (medroxyprogesterone). From these studies six conclusions were drawn:

- Increased risk of cardiovascular disease with 5mgs DES
- Orchidectomy and DES no better than orchidectomy alone
- Equivalent cancer control with 1mg and 5mg DES
- Premarin and Provera were no better than DES
- Significantly decreased risk of cardiovascular deaths with 1mg DES
- When to give treatment was dependent on patient characteristics, a reanalysis showed only those patients with high risk disease appeared to benefit from immediate treatment.

At the end of the 1960s, three separate groups reported the isolation of the androgen receptor in the rat prostate (Liao, Bruchovsky and Mainwaring). This meant that there was now a protein target against which drug companies could hope to produce new drugs that specifically blocked the action of the male hormone in men and hopefully would cause shrinkage of prostate cancer without the side effects current therapies produced. These developments came to fruition during the 1980s when a great many other things changed.

The classical description of the pathology of prostate cancer followed the pattern of most cancers in which well, moderately, and poorly differentiated types were identified. In prostate, as with other cancers, 'if it looked good, it did good, and if it looked bad, it did bad.' In 1967 Gleason proposed a modified way of characterising prostate cancer. He found that if he looked carefully, there were often two patterns, at relatively low-powered magnification, if they were the same that determined prognosis, but if two were present, then the more aggressive, even if quite small, determined prognosis. His scoring system went from 1 to 5, so that a score could be awarded; the higher the number, the more aggressive the tumour.

In 1956 Whitmore described a simple clinical system for classifying prostate cancer based on rectal examination.

A, No tumour was palpable.
B, Palpable tumour which was confined to the prostate.
C, A tumour that could be felt beyond the boundary of the prostate.

D, Usually similar to C but with evidence from x-rays that the cancer had spread.

During the 1960s Hugh Jewett at Johns Hopkins refined this system especially with respect to A and B, which was subsequently shown to have great clinical usage. A was still no palpable tumour but divided into A1 and A2 depending on the volume of cancer which had been found, usually following surgery for what was thought to be benign disease.

But a clinical difference between B1 and B2 was defined. A small nodule or disease was on one lobe of the prostate only against B2, which signifies a larger volume in one lobe or present in both lobes. This is a clinical system, i.e. what a surgeon feels, and although it became more refined, with a,b,c, suffixes, it was entirely subjective. What appears to have stood the test of time with sophisticated, modern imaging, is that the B1 nodule, the 1cm one, still carries a good prognosis but the German clinical study in the 70s could not show a clinical benefit to patients because of the subjectivity of what is a 1cm nodule. The presence of disease in both lobes seemed to have a significant prognostic value.

In retrospective studies of the Johns Hopkins experience, with cases going back to Hugh Young's later ones, Jewett determined several important outcomes as related to surgery.

-- First, he found that no patient with high-risk disease survived 15 years.

-- Second, only 5% of patients with seminal vesicle invasion survived 15 years.

-- Third, only 16% of patients with B1 disease had seminal vesicle invasion, and this group, albeit only in the few dozens, appeared to do well with surgery, and of equal interest, better as a group than A2 disease. If no treatment was given to A1 disease, there was no record that these patients ever developed metastases.

These results were neatly summarised in a joint paper by Patrick Walsh and Hugh Jewett in 1980, reviewing the Hopkins data. It was clear from their analysis that only a small cohort of patients benefitted from surgery, from their figures; the problem was how to find them. In Germany a form of screening in which men having their annual medicals had a documented rectal examination to see if pick up rates could be improved, but this did not occur, and in 2002 when this study was repeated, now with the benefits of PSA and biopsy readily available, diagnoses based on clinical examination alone had similar poor pick-up rates to those from the 1970s.

The situation, then, appeared settled. A small discrete group of patients may gain a cure from surgery, but most appeared to do as well with radiation therapy. Palliative therapy with hormone therapy or its equivalent was very effective even in the most advanced of cases, with active life being prolonged for a couple of years at worst. When hormones failed attempts had been made to see if a secondary hormone response was possible, usually by using either hormones if an orchidectomy had been the primary treatment, and *vice versa*, and some cases of bilateral adrenalectomy, and even the removal of the pituitary, hypophysectomy, related temporary responses in pain control, or acid phosphatase decline.

However, it remained predominantly a disease of the older man, and younger men had much more serious problems such as the mortality from cardiovascular disease, scything them down in their fifties to be too concerned about a disease of the over-seventies.

Things were about to change, however.

4. Changes

When Patrick Walsh took up his post at Johns Hopkins, the home of the operation, he found no radical prostatectomies being performed. As we have seen, review of the Hopkins data appeared to show a small, but distinct group of men that could, or should be cured of their cancer by surgery. The problem he defined was in the unacceptable complications of impotence and incontinence in relatively young men. He set out to devise an operation that secured a potential cure with fewer complications.

After careful anatomical reviews against a background of the earlier work of Gil-Vernet, and in collaboration with the Dutch anatomist Donker, he identified three principal areas of attention. First, the large complex of veins on top of the prostate (Santorini's plexus, now more prosaically, the dorsal vein complex) needed to be secured early. Next, the neurovascular bundles running alongside the prostate capsule needed identifying, and preserving; and once the prostate was removed, following Jewett's recommendation, a more accurate re-joining of the urethra and bladder neck, the hockey stick approach, improved the chances of urinary continence (Walsh 1982). The first anatomic, radical prostatectomy was performed in March 1982, and by the end of the decade the Hopkins series was nearly a thousand, though as will be appreciated, the average length of follow up was less than five years, and Jewett had always felt that 15 years was the minimum necessary to see that the operation was changing the outcome of the disease.

Several other groups in the USA, Catalona in St Louis, Myers at the Mayo Clinic and others produced large series of patients following Walsh's technique, with small variations; indeed over the course of the next twenty years Walsh himself introduced up to a dozen small changes in points of technique. What was indisputable was that both the continence and potency rates were far better than any previously reported series and the practicality of the procedure was that it could be exported to other centres where expert surgeons replicated the results.

Surgical procedures should be a reliably deliverable therapy, with the same predicted outcomes as when patients take drugs. It is possible to tip the results in a favourable direction because of selection bias, but

Walsh's cohort of younger patients (fit and aged below seventy, with small volume, localised disease) was precisely the group that seemed to have the best chance of a cure of their prostate cancer. All of these cases, while emphasising the greatly improved fall in complications, remained more cautious about the oncological effect. Although the cases were carefully selected, inevitably because of the multiplicity of tumours found in many prostates, some of these were high risk, and predictably did less well that the intermediate- and low-risk patients. At this stage, everyone was talking about 'potentially curable' cases.

It was not only the rationale for treating this group of patients provided by the retrospective review of the Hopkins data, but the consensus of cancer development at this time; and the basis for surgical treatment of all tumours was that it always started small, and enlarged and became more aggressive with enlargement, until it was large enough to breach the confines of its originating organ, to spread to local tissue, and the lymph glands that drained this organ, and eventually to enter the blood stream and appear in other parts of the body, frequently the lungs or liver, as metastases. Prostate cancer was considered unusual in several ways. Firstly, alongside lung, breast, kidney and thyroid, it had a propensity to spread to bone, and secondly, the lesions in the bone were sclerotic (hard or dense), unlike the other cancers whose bone lesions were lytic (destroyed; literally there were holes in the bones), although sometimes dense lesions could form in these. Only occasionally did prostate cancer present just with lymph gland enlargement, and clinical experience showed that these respond very well to hormone treatment and more predictably, with often complete disappearance of the enlarged glands.

The work-up of the patient at this time combined clinical examination of the prostate, x-rays and bone scans, together with acid and alkaline phosphatase. All investigations including general ones to exclude anaemia, renal and liver abnormalities had to be normal, and the patient fit for major surgery. This is how, inevitably, selection bias creeps in. High blood pressure, heart or lung disease made it easy to exclude the patient because of the surgical risks and recommend radiation therapy. The patients available for surgery almost selected themselves.

I became acquainted with patient B who, having rejected Watchful Waiting as the treatment for his prostate cancer, had a radical prostatectomy in one of the major US centres in the 1990s when the procedure was well established and almost routine. He was a spry, wiry, 58-year-old with no other medical problems. He was amazed to find himself the oldest patient on the ward awaiting the procedure, which was expertly delivered, and he rapidly became continent and had normal erections. I asked what prognosis he had been offered, 12 years without disease problems, but a bit hazy after that, although it was likely to be fine. What was the Watchful Waiting prognosis you were offered? I enquired. Oh, that was 12 years as well. Even at this time, in the best centres, the words 'potentially curative' were still operative.

An interesting side light on selection bias has been shown recently in the UK. When it was proposed to publish individual surgeons' figures, surgeons were concerned, not that their figures were bad, but that it would induce defensive practice, and only 'easy' cases would be taken on, giving predictably good outcomes. Fortunately, as the cardiovascular surgeons, and most recently the coloproctology surgeons have shown, this has not been the case, and indeed the difficulty of the cases has increased (Alderson, PRCS 2018).

Although the long-term cancer cure rates still remained to be determined, radical prostatectomy as a procedure had progressed significantly. There were still problems, the procedure was difficult, and as experience grew, more patients were encountered that still appeared to have their cancer confined to one side, but it had begun to encroach on the neurovascular bundle, which had to be sacrificed to leave a margin of clearance from tumour cells. However, even with only one bundle intact, men were able to regain erections.

The procedure was refined, all that was needed now was a way of finding more prostate cancer patients earlier.

Prostate Specific Antigen (PSA)

PSA is a protein secreted by prostate cells into the prostatic fluid. It causes unclotting of semen clumps, thus promoting active and free sperm movement. It has been described by a number of scientists from the late 1960s (Flocks, Ablin amongst them), but the work of Wang (1979) demonstrated PSA in the serum, and thereafter work by Stamey in Stanford began to elucidate its usefulness in prostate cancer and its role as a marker for prostate cancer (Stamey 1987). The first commercial serum

PSA test (The Hybritech Tandem-R PSA test) was released in 1986, and its reference range for normals of less than 4ng/ml was based on their licensing study which found 5 of 472 men who were apparently healthy and were not known to have prostate cancer, had a total PSA above 4ng/ml, although the upper limit of normal was much less than 4.0ng/ml.

Its initial licence, approved by the FDA (Food and Drugs Administration) in the USA, was as a marker of prostate cancer activity, and commenced in 1986. It proved to be much more sensitive than the existing acid phosphatase, although it didn't always convey as much information as using both acid and alkaline phosphatase. In 1991 the American Cancer Society National Prostate Cancer Project reported findings on the detection of early prostate cancer in 2,425 men (Mettlin 1991). This led in 1994 the FDA to approve the test in conjunction with a digital rectal examination (DRE, the old rectal exam polyphonically updated) to screen asymptomatic men for prostate cancer. The rest of the world soon followed this example, some a little more laggardly than others, whether they had a single- or multiple-payer health care system being directly related to the speed or otherwise of its adoption. (The UK NHS is still currently a single-payer system).

In 1968 Wilson and Junger set out clear criteria in their principles and practice of screening for disease. As genomic screening became a real probability, there was a slightly modified version published in 2008, but they are broadly similar. Looking at them carefully will help to explain why PSA screening has been so controversial.

1. The condition should be an important health problem.
2. There should be a proven treatment for the condition.
3. Facilities for diagnosis and treatment should be available.
4. There should be a latent phase of the disease.
5. There should be a test or examination for the condition.
6. The test should be acceptable to the population.
7. The natural history of the disease should be adequately understood.
8. There should be an agreed policy on whom to treat.
9. The total cost of finding a case should be economically balanced in relation to medical expenditure as a whole.
10. Case finding should be a continuous process, not just a once and for all project.

PSA failed right at the beginning of its use because it was unable to tell which men, the majority, did not have prostate cancer. It rapidly became apparent that the range, whilst helpful in monitoring known cases of prostate cancer, even when used in combination with TRUS (trans rectal ultrasound and biopsy) could only identify if the disease was present but in no way reassure those with a negative biopsy that no disease existed. The recommendation had to be repeat biopsies, although the intervals were not known, and the level of the blood test to be used as a guide became more difficult when up to 20% of cancers being found were in what was alleged to be the normal range. Nor were biopsies a benign process. Anywhere up to 4% of patients developed infections requiring courses of antibiotics, 1% needed hospitalisation, and there were a number of deaths from generalised sepsis. Given that the initial estimates were that perhaps one in a thousand men undergoing PSA testing would be found to have prostate cancer and was potentially curable, it looked very much as though the deaths from the investigation would just about balance out the lives saved. Furthermore as we look through these criteria it was obvious that screening between 50 and 69 must uncover a large number of latent cancers which we understood would do no harm, but we had not yet worked out any method to distinguish those of low aggressiveness from those over the next ten years that would become dangerous and life threatening. Invariably clinicians faced with the onslaught of men with marginally elevated PSA levels compromised.

Patient C had just turned 50 when, as he helped his father to his final radiotherapy session for his prostate cancer, was helpfully told by a nurse that he should have a PSA test. This he did and it came back at 4.8ng/ml. His GP, an experienced man, recommended he repeat it in three months. It was then 4.7, so he was referred. I spent a long time going over with him what we knew and what was now becoming worldwide policy, especially that we suspected that a familial history did place the patient at risk. Well, he said, that was all very well, but his wife had just been diagnosed with breast cancer, having had her biopsy confirmed and was booked for surgery and any subsequent treatment. He felt they couldn't cope with two cancers simultaneously; was there anything else they could do? I said that there was some evidence that the speed of rise of the PSA could indicate activity and cause for concern, why didn't we agree on a very conservative scheme of serial PSA measurement, and if the value crossed the threshold he would go off and have his scan and biopsy. We talked about the psychological burden he would carry, but he felt worrying about his wife would keep him occupied. Over the next few years, with measurements initially at three months, but then mostly six monthly the PSA rose incrementally until five and a half years later it passed our agreed threshold of 6.0ng/ml, a purely arbitrary value. Well, he said, that's good. My wife has just got the all clear and she wants me to know what's going on and get it treated if it is a cancer. He had a biopsy, and it was a Gleason3+4 cancer. Although I explained we could still watch this and see if it rose further so that the side effects of surgery and radiation therapy could be avoided, he felt his wife expected him to have his cancer treated, even though we both knew it had been there for at least six years by this time, and had not just turned up. He opted to have surgery and had some post-operative urinary and potency complic-ations, the latter not resolving even when viagra, which had just ap-peared, was used. His PSA has remained undetectable into his seventies and must represent, in all probability, a definite cure from intervention. What I learnt is that speed is not of the essence in this tumour.

Over the next two decades many thousands of papers were written about PSA, some of which will be reviewed in due course, and further elaboration of PSA, free PSA and total PSA, the remainder being bound to a protein still could not get over the basic problem that a lower limit could not be assigned below which no patient had prostate cancer. In an enthusiastic rush reducing the upper value from 4.0ng/ml to 3ng/ml mar-ginally increased the pick-up rate of cancer, but what types of cancers were picked up awaited a longer follow-up period than we would ima-gine.

New Imagining

The first transrectal ultrasound machine to be developed required the pa-tient to sit on a metal chair, a circular portion of the middle of which had been removed, and through which the ultrasound probe rose and entered the rectum; the image was recorded on a screen adjacent. Brian Peeling, who was the first UK urologist to use the machine which came from Ja-pan, recorded that patients were not at all enamoured of it, with several doughty Welshmen telling him they would be b-----ed if they were going to sit on that.

However, the technology moved swiftly forward, and soon hand-held ultrasound machines became available, with the added benefit that biopsies could be taken through them. Hitherto, urologists had used biopsy needles guided by the finger to take biopsies, and had largely given up the transrectal route because of the risk of infections, instead steadying the prostate via the rectum and passing the needle into the prostate via the perineum, historically always the favoured route to avoid infection.

Almost simultaneously with a possible marker of prostate cancer, an imaging system, portable and therefore readily usable in the clinic, became available.

The discovery of x-ray computer tomography (CT scanning) enabled much more detailed images that were three dimensional to be taken, helping to stage patients more efficiently, but it did not really help with a change in the delivery of radiation therapy, which up to the early 1990s remained two dimensional, although the linacs improved and the amount of radiation was increased that was delivered to the prostate.

The use of the technetium radioactive isotope which preferentially homed in on diseased bones, enable a faster and more accurate assessment of the presence, or otherwise, of bony metastases, than the older skeletal survey, which to be accurate had to x-ray every bone.

It now meant it was possible to confirm both the effectiveness of treatment as with the fall of PSA the lesions highlighted by the bone scan also faded in parallel with them.

New Drugs

Once the androgen receptor had been characterised it was possible for scientists in pharmaceutical companies to try to fashion drugs that could block the receptor and stop it working. It was hoped that these new agents would be just as effective as orchidectomy and stilboestrol, without the unpleasant side effects patients suffered from either treatment. Cyproterone acetate was one of the first to be used but it combined a progesterone as well as a pure anti-androgen function, as progesterone in the late 1960s and early 1970s was thought to add a benefit. Flutamide was the first pure anti-androgen, to be followed by nilutamide, and then bicalutamide, which has appeared to have the lowest side effects profile over time.

An interesting example of a drug looking for a home was the development of LH-RH agonists. In 1971 Andrew Schally showed how hormones that were produced in the hypothalamus part of the brain, LH (luteinising hormone) releasing hormone (RH) travelled to the pituitary and by stopping the release of LH prevented, downstream, the production of testosterone, although his early studies showed this in oestrogens, as it was hoped this mechanism would prove to be a useful female contraceptive. Things along this line didn't work out, not least because in its early phase an injection needed to be given on a daily basis. By very skilled chemical engineering, the drug was produced that as a small pellet could be injected subcutaneously and slowly released the active agent regularly over 28 days, which then stretched to three, and then six months. Because it was an agonist it initially produced a 'flare' or rise in testosterone production before the level of testosterone fell. Anti-androgens were handily available to cover this in the week or so it occurred.

A number of large, randomised trials took place seeking to show that these new agents were equivalent to orchidectomy. By and large this appeared broadly so, although none could show sustained superiority, and they brought their own complications, plus the new, potentially serious one, in men with metastases, of activating the tumour during the 'flare' before control was achieved.

Such sophistication, naturally, did not come cheap; how then was an expensive agent that did no better than the old standbys, and without precautions could bring more problems, replace the existing treatments? There was no virtue, as single-payer systems succumbed just as readily as multi-payer ones.

If the fee for an orchidectomy was, say, $400, and practitioners were offered $50 a month for giving the injection, it is a no brainer, given the survival of even the worst affected prostate cancer patient with metastases, 18 months to two years to see how preference could easily shift, and it only needed a few experts to dismiss oestrogen treatment, which only cost pence, as 'of historic interest' only for the circle to be neatly squared. In single-payer countries such as the UK, mysteriously stories appeared in both the medical and lay press excoriating the possibly unethical practice of castration (orchidectomy), and lamenting that patients were being denied modern treatment, for patients to demand the new drug. Curiously, whilst the case was wildly against the barbaric and medieval practice of 'surgical castration', medical castration which the new drugs offered was seen as more 'gentlemanly' and with such attribution, more costly.

Also, many urological departments were engaged in putting patients into clinical trials, with the drug, in this era being provided by the company until the drug obtained a licence, that the basics of consumer demand was there. In the UK a payment for giving the injections in the community also helped to make its reception positive.

As we shall see, despite all the activity, no new insights were gained that superseded those already promulgated by Huggins; they work, they don't appear to cure, prolonged responses may happen, but we can only vaguely predict .There could have been some leger-de-main in this process, but neither the clinicians nor the pharmaceutical companies had expected or were prepared for what was to happen when PSA was let loose on an unsuspecting world as a marker for detecting symptomatic, early stage prostate cancer.

5. The Rise

As more of the major American centres adopted the Walsh modifications of radical prostatectomy, and obtained outcomes in the way of continence and the preservation of erectile function much better than the older surgical methods, some began to push for the use of PSA as initially a case-finding tool; that is, using it in all men who came to a urologist with urinary symptoms, and then to suggest that it be utilised as a possible screening test (Stamey 1987). Figures from the USA show a steady rise in the number of cases in the USA from 100,000 at the beginning of the 1980s to 140,000 at the end. The rapid incorporation of transrectal ultrasound and biopsy made this readily available, and increasingly 'awareness weeks' following those of breast and colon cancer brought the message, greatly simplified, of course, of a test, a treatment and a cure.

In the early 1990s in the USA the incidence reached over a quarter of a million a year just before the FDA in 1994 licensed PSA to be used as a screening tool. Thereafter, the incident figure remained at least twice that of the early 1980s figure, and in recent years has fallen back to 160,000 to 180,000. The death rates also rose, although slightly behind that of the incidence to a maximum figure of just over 40,000 before dropping back to the 1980s death toll in numbers of 30,000. These figures appeared independent of any treatment given.

The availability of PSA fuelled the rise, but there was no subsequent significant rise when PSA was recommended as a screening test, possibly because anyone who was eligible had already had the PSA done. The awareness campaigns were remarkably successful; analysis of Dutch incidence rates suggests that their early 1990s surge was wholly attributable to increased awareness and the availability of transrectal ultrasound, and it was possible to identify a further spike in 2001 (Cremers), when PSA screening became widely possible.

Once the PSA was found to be elevated, a biopsy was recommended. If prostate cancer was identified, then the patients, not unreasonably, expected treatment. They had a cancer, it had been found when it was still not giving symptoms, it could only get worse, so said the popular conception of cancer, and no one went into the almost Jesuitical discussions that might have been necessary to explain absolute and relative risk; and anyway if you would not carry out treatment, in the USA and elsewhere, you need only walk down the street to find someone who would do the right thing.

The complications from a radical prostatectomy had, in the specialist centres, come down to levels which were acceptable to the patients, especially as many thought that without treatment they would succumb to cancer in the next year or so at most. There was no general misinformation. Many clinicians viewed these small volume, low-risk cases as exactly those Walsh had described whose removal would lead to a cure, and equated having the operation as a cure, and not having the procedure as being neglectful.

Transrectal biopsy proved to be a poor predictor of outcome. There were no uniform images that consistently showed an abnormality; given that the procedure was operator dependent, images changed, and recommendations to take more specimens were given. Even so, review of the operative specimen often demonstrated many more lesions than had been thought, sometimes with more aggressive pathology, and sometimes little was found.

A distressing case, Patient D, was brought to our pathology meeting by a colleague from another hospital. Unequivocally, the biopsy specimen showed a part of one of six cores to have, what everyone agreed to be prostate cancer. The local pathologist and our referral centre pathologist had scoured the specimen, to no avail. Not a single further piece of tumour was found. By chance the whole tumour had been removed by the needle at biopsy. Reflection, hindsight is always 100% correct; most people felt that this had been a sledgehammer to crack a nut. As we will discuss in the next chapter, the experts reported that results which still left men impotent and with continence problems were not directly transferrable.

In the major departments in the USA prostate cancer seemed the only disease being treated. One of my trainees visited one of these in the mid-1990s. Although only there for a couple of weeks, and very keen to learn all about prostatectomy from a world expert, he was surprised to find himself acting as first assistant to the big chief himself and maintained that situation throughout his stay. He was, and is, an extremely good surgeon, so the patients were definitely advantaged, but he saw more prostatectomies carried out in his couple of weeks there than had been done in the whole of the UK in that period.

Another problem that presented itself affected my own practice. Based on the Hopkins figures, the standard of care of an incidental, less than 5% of tissue from a resection of the prostate for urinary problems, the patient was told that a small amount of cancer had been found but that it was unlikely to cause any future problems and no treatment was advised. Towards the end of the 1990s when PSA testing became more widely available in the UK, several of my patients, now in their late 70s or early 80s had had PSA tests; all were found to be above the level of 4ng/ml, and back they came to see me. Although clinically they appeared fine, I dutifully arranged TRUS (transrectal ultrasound and biopsy). All came back positive, but on careful pathological review, all had the same looking tumour that they had had ten or fifteen years ago. I strongly urged them to do nothing, and none, I'm pleased to say, came to any sub-sequent harm from their 'touch of prostate cancer'.

Approaching 150,000 radical prostatectomies a year were carried out in the next few years in the USA, and after a slower start most high-income countries followed suit. It was obvious to many that the scientific basis on which the rationale for this activity was vanishingly small, based on a few hundred retrospective cases at best and that RCTs (randomised controlled trials) about the effectiveness of screening, and contemporary treatment were necessary.

The first into the field was the Quebec Randomised Control Trial which reported in 1999. This involved 46,193 men aged 45-80, who were randomised to no screening, or screening with PSA and DRE (rectal ex-amination, the D stands for digital, a given for most people). A PSA level above 3ng/ml led to a TRUS and biopsy. Follow up thereafter was by PSA alone. The end point was prostate cancer mortality, and the follow up period was 7 years. 137 deaths were reported in the 38,056 un-screened patients and only 5 among the screened population of 8,137. Without resorting to statistics, and to the obvious advantage to the screened individuals. However, the analysis was done as per an observa-tional study, not as a RCT as it should have been. This introduced several biases which could not be calculated and undoubtedly left the result overestimating the benefits of screening. Moreover, Walsh and Jewett had both felt 15 years to be the minimum follow up necessary in these patients, and expert opinion worldwide agreed; given the natural history of the disease, this was the minimum follow up acceptable.

The PLCO (prostate, lung, colon, ovary) screening trial was a US study involving multiple institutions, looking at these significant cancers. Breast had already developed its own screening regime based on mammography. In the prostate arm, 76,693 men between 55 and 74 were randomly assigned to annual screening with PSA and DRE using 4ng/ml as the cut-off value and an abnormal feeling prostate as indications to go forward for further tests. The control arm had usual care. This study reported on cancer incidence, cancer-specific mortality, all-cause mortality, and accurate cancer staging when found. This was one of the few studies that had a high compliance rate in adhering to the protocol, and in getting the targeted patient accrual. However, it also initially reported at seven years, and essentially showed no difference between the screened and non-screened populations. This weakness was addressed with a later report on 13 year follow up, and although more cancers were found in the screened arm, the cancer-specific mortality was the same. This trial, despite its virtues, was also criticised as many men in the unscreened arm had also had annual PSA tests, their usual practice, so that some of those assigned to the unscreened arms had in effect been screened at least once off trial, and worrisome cases dealt with, so the pool of controls was undermined. Again it was difficult to assess how serious this had been (Andriole 2009). An updated review in 2017 will be discussed later.

The European RCT (ERSPC) was co-ordinated by Fritz Schroeder, Professor of Urology in Rotterdam, and involved 182,160 men from a number of countries, but most patients came from the Low Countries and Scandinavia. The PSA cut off was between 2.5 and 4 with most countries using 3.0 as their level. A brief summary of a great deal of work in the 162,243 men aged 55-69 at 11 years follow up showed that the prostate cancer mortality was lower, by a fifth, and the reduction of metastatic disease in the screened group was two- fifths. All-cause mortality was not changed, i.e. the screened group did not live longer but possibly died of something else in the long follow up period of 11 years. A further analysis by Schroeder in 2012 showed consolidation of these initially reported results.

This study was also criticised for a number of aspects and although showing some benefit possibly did not demonstrate clear blue water between the treated and non-treated and confirmed the concern of many by now that overdiagnosis and overtreatment were probably causing more problems than the screening solved. This will be discussed chronologically as these worries crystallised.

A final screening study was associated with a randomised trial of therapies (ProTech) and was carried out in the UK. The CAP part of the study was a one-off PSA testing from general practitioner lists in 9 participating areas of the UK. Practices were randomised for men to receive or not an invitation for a PSA test. 415,357 men were included in this study; half were invited for the blood test, and approximately two-thirds of these had a valid test. Those found to have prostate cancer were then invited to take part in the clinical studies. They also essentially showed no benefit in reducing cancer-specific or overall mortality (2017 Donovan).

It was also realised that properly conducted clinical trials were essential, not easy to try to identify the patients, based on the Hopkins figures who would benefit from early intervention. Three groups organised such prospective randomised trials: the American based PIVOT study which randomised 731 men between November 1994 and June 2000, into either surgery or watchful waiting (i.e. no intervention); the Scan4 study, which incorporated patients from the countries of this area – between 1989 and 1995, they randomised 695 patients to either surgery or watchful waiting; and finally the UK ProTech study had completed its recruitment in 2004 of patients from the CAP screening study when just under 1,700 patients were randomised to either surgery, R/T, or active surveillance (this, as we will see, had taken the place of watchful waiting and implied a greater possibility of intervention for these patients).

All these studies reported 10-year outcomes between 2013 and 2016 and we will examine these in their due place. It must be realised that no one felt they could wait for even the ten year results of these trials as there were patients to treat, and all, realistically could not be put into trials. Best judgement on the evidence at the time was all that could be provided, but it is striking in the reports of the time how the cautious word 'potentially curable' used by the surgical pioneers seemed to have fallen out of use, although when challenged to state who was actually being cured here, the reply came that longer follow up was, obviously, necessary.

6. Consequences

Being a surgeon is a great privilege and performing surgery cures people of many ailments promptly and permanently. To paraphrase the German military philosopher, Clausewitz, 'it is a very simple thing, but even the simplest thing is very difficult.'

In essence surgery repairs, restructures, or removes disease. It is with the last, removal, that we are most concerned when discussing prostate cancer. It is probably easier to understand the basic concept when thinking of breast cancer. An abnormal lump is found and is removed with sufficient margin to be completely clear of any tumour. Concepts and fashions change, but within living memory it was considered vital, when dealing with breast cancer, to remove everything down to the rib cage, the super-radical mastectomy, whereas now in many cases removing the lump with a margin is deemed sufficient. I realise this is simplistic, but it emphasises that the concepts don't change but how it is achieved can be radically different.

Therefore, the prostate needs removing, with a margin of normal tissue to ensure clearance. This was perfectly executed by Young, but with all his patients impotent, and a third permanently incontinent. For a benefit in only a small number of patients, the side effects were felt to be far worse than the disease. As we have seen, Walsh's great contribution was to identify the nerves that may be spared, and thus help to maintain erections and continence, but also to reconstruct the bladder neck so that the chance of incontinence was reduced.

In a cohort of young patients (2000) who were potent before having their radical prostatectomy by Walsh, 86% retained their potency but a third did need viagra (this became available in 1997) and 93% were totally dry and fully continent. However, most surgeons were not Patrick Walsh.

Surgery, as a treatment, should be deliverable consistently as to outcome and within a relatively narrow range, with regard to complications. No amount of repetition can eliminate the chance of a complication following a surgical procedure. In the more muscular times when I trained, if you hadn't seen a complication with any procedure, you were assured that it was because you hadn't done enough rather than due to your exceptional skill.

Donald Rumsfeld, the US Defence Secretary in the Bush administration, was ridiculed for his trying to define problems. The known, knowns, the known /unknowns, and then the unknown/unknowns; surgeons can identify with this categorisation easily. This is why surgeons have a way of doing something which they carefully follow, to ensure patient safety, and get very upset if disturbed or put off their stroke. Changing the environment by non-clinicians puts patients at considerable risk; there is no routine operation. All patients having their operations are dealt with very carefully. This was illustrated in a neat trial published in the *Lancet* (1850) when propranolol, a beta blocker, was first being used. A group of surgeons performing an inguinal hernia repair had their pulse monitored just before commencing the operation. All surgeons, whatever their age or experience, had elevation of their pulse rates to over 100, which the propranolol would help settle. Few surgeons would take these pills, preferring the adrenaline rush to keep them alert and working well.

Walsh's series, which shows excellent results, does, however, demonstrate another problem surgeons are very aware of. Selection bias. In fairness to Walsh, this is showing what his procedure with careful selection of patients can achieve, and his more general case mix still has good results, but many surgeons have a cause for worry if individual data is published, and have concerns that sanctions on outcomes would restrict possibly life-saving operations being denied patients because they represent a higher risk and could make the figures look bad. Fortunately, as the UK coloproctology surgeons have demonstrated, if agreed inclusion criteria are adhered to, and the operation performed for the correct indication, then, as it should, outcomes are predictably delivered, and over time the results collectively improve, but none is without some complications.

Similarly, the admirable UK GIRFT (get it right first time) campaign, which will pull up the average by adopting the best measures of many practitioners, but again a risk-free, complication-free practice is unobtainable. The outcomes must be based on what is deliverable by the average surgeon. This should be very good, but it is foolish to base desired outcomes on the best. If a surgical procedure can only be done by one surgeon in one hospital, then he/she should do all the cases, or the procedure still needs work on it in order to travel.

This is a slightly circuitous route to look at surgical outcomes when everyone was doing radical prostatectomies. Fowler et al (1993) first published their patient-reported outcomes (PROMS) in 1990 and then updated them in 1993. The complications of radical prostatectomy were not like those of the major centres at all; indeed, they were more like those from the earlier era, with the majority of patients reporting both impotence and varying degrees of incontinence. High-risk cases had been eschewed, and many were small-volume, low-risk cancers that would not have imposed any risk to life. It was a rude awakening, and reality check.

There was really no alternative to patients demanding treatment now their cancer had been found. Fowler and colleagues published data on patient-reported outcomes on radiotherapy side effects in 1996 which showed that these were not trivial and brought in bowel disturbances to add to urine incontinence and impotence. In 2000 a further study from this group examined men who had or had not been put onto ADT (androgen deprivation therapy), and found that their urinary incontinence rate was similar, being about 25%, but even in the non-drug taking group impotence was still above 50%. There had obviously been an improvement in operative technique, but both complications remained relatively high. To bring this up to date, and which will be discussed later, a review in JAMA in 2018 estimated, in general, that 1:5 men had urinary issues post radical prostatectomy, and 2:3 were impotent. This did not take account as to how many were impotent before the operation.

In 1999 the Hopkins groups published data on 304 men who had developed a PSA rise after radical prostatectomy, where by common consent, if the prostate had been removed, then the PSA should be unmeasurable, and any recurrence of PSA measurement meant that the disease was present, although it was not able to differentiate whether this was local or distant spread. The differentiation had become important, for as pathologists became familiar with the deluge of specimens, it became obvious that some showed the tumour to be enclosed by normal tissue whilst others (margin positive) had tumour right up to the edge of the specimen. It was then a dilemma as to whether local radiation therapy should be given or whether they should be watched or started on hormone (ADT) therapy.

The Hopkins results offered some reassurance, but this data was only available long after decisions had had to be made on men with similar problems. 34% of the group developed demonstrable metastases, and 43% of these, so about a quarter of the total 304 died of prostate cancer, after a median follow-up time of 5.3 years. In the group as a whole it took a median of 8 years to develop metastases, and a further 5 years to die from the disease. The difference in the two results given is that some of the tumours will have been found to have highly aggressive tumours, which would be as predicted; neither the surgery nor subsequent hormone treatment imposed more than a delay in the inevitable outcome.

Many surgeons in the USA were confronted as to what to do with patients having a rising PSA following surgery. The rest of the world was a few years behind and could have learnt from their experience; they didn't appear to.

Having offered a patient a cure, often after soliciting them to have a 'life-saving blood test', it was extremely difficult, if not impossible, to then recommend that we just watch this, and if it goes to bone and causes symptoms, we will then start the patient on ADT. Whether giving hormones early did anything for patients was a moot point, pathologically, but it did drive the PSA down, which was good for morale and not to be disparaged. Inevitably the patients got side effects from long-term hormone treatment, but in some the PSA began to rise again. More worryingly, bone scans and body scans could not show that there were any demonstrable metastases. Just in time for the millennium a new disease, hormone resistant nonmetastatic prostate cancer was born. A wholly iatrogenic disease (medically induced). What could be done?

Well, firstly it was always worthwhile trying different hormones, which although not as effective in the secondary phase, did stabilise PSA values and sometimes drove them down. There was, however, at this time no chemotherapeutic agents that showed any benefit in prostate cancer. Some relief was obtained with steroids, but these patients represented a very difficult management problem mostly because they had been asymptomatic before they started and had believed, whatever they had been told, that an early diagnosis and an operation would give them a cure, so they would not suffer from prostate cancer.

This is the first quite distinct group who lost control of their lives. At this stage it was no use telling them that an option would have been to do nothing, as they were unlikely to be any worse off, and may well not have had treatment for some time. Elsewhere in the world were men who had prostate cancer, and no one had found it for them. They therefore led their lives completely unaware of their potential difficulties. They could have missed out on a cure, but they certainly would have a complication-free life of many years before having a diagnosis and commencing on what everyone knew from the past was palliative treatment.

Meanwhile new technology and the obvious complications of the surgery had brought into focus alternatives for primary treatment.

7. Competition

The further development of CT scanning and its integration into radiotherapy planning led in the early 1990s to the creation of three-dimensional conformal radiotherapy (3D-CRT). Put simply, this was a method that allowed radiotherapy beams to be shaped to conform with the shape of a tumour on the patient's planning scan. Conforming the beams helped to maximise the amount of radiation delivered to the tumour, whilst minimising the radiation delivered to the pelvic organs and thus minimising the side effects of treatment. A RCT (Dearnaley 1999) showed that using this technique with conventional radiotherapy using the standard dose, 64Gy, showed a significant reduction in proctitis, especially with no change in the ability to exert disease control.

Two further changes occurred that enabled higher doses of radiation to be given to the prostate while keeping the side effects within tolerable bounds. A more advanced form of 3D-CRT led to the creation of 'intensity modulated radiotherapy (IMRT)'; this allowed more beams to be used, and this was followed by dose escalation in which consistently higher doses of radiation therapy were delivered with the same side effects profile. A series of RCTs showed that the dose could be upped from 64 to 86, although most aimed for between 74 and 78 Gy and these reported improved freedom from biochemical or clinical failure. A US study showed the benefits to be 78% versus 59%. Importantly, high-risk patients were involved, and although not doing so well as lower categories, control for more than half was exhibited for five or more years.

The most significant advance, however, was in locally advanced disease, where the chances of lymph gland involvement was high, and the chances of them all being in the radiation field was low. The EORTC (European Organisation for Research and Treatment of Cancer,) led by Michel Bolla from Grenoble (2002), conducted a study in which all patients received 70 Gy, but half also went on to 3 years ADT starting on the first day of radiation. The 10-year disease-free survival of this significantly at-risk group was 22.7% in the radiation arm alone, and 47% in the combined treatment arm. More compelling, and of greater relevance for patients was that the overall survival in the radiation-alone group was 39.8% whilst in the combined arm, 58.1%. Shortly after an American RTC showed that the same effects could be obtained with six months of ADT (D'Amico, 2004).

In 2009 a Scandinavian study showed the superiority of the combination against ADT alone, the findings confirmed by a large inter-group study which reported in 2011.That the combination should be used in high- risk patients appears unarguable, but the duration of the hormones remains a matter of debate. The conservatives support longer because cancer cells are still being killed up to 18 months after treatment, and this needs covering. The more radical support the shorter course on the principle that the best has been obtained by six months, and that in this high-risk group there is a good chance that the hormones will be needed for further palliative treatment. Patients do have a choice here when discussing matters with their own doctor.

Patient E is a friend more than an acquaintance. At the age of 83 he came to see me, and we ended up with a diagnosis of prostate cancer, PSA 16.0 ng/ml, and Gleason 8. Well, I said, this is where we are, what is your ambition for the next decade? And the rest, he told me. My ambition is to be 100. Right. As so often happens, talk of how studies were doing, especially ones that were giving a positive result, it seemed were around long before a paper was published. Our department and radiotherapists had participated in the EORTC study and so it was possible to treat as per protocol but off study which had closed to recruitment. Patient E also chose the shorter drug regime having carefully read all the side effects. He is now four years from his goal but has had to have several courses of hormones, but because of the profound exhaustion they induce, is always keen, once his PSA has fallen, to stop all drugs. Despite his readiness to take part in research projects we have no idea how he does it.

But there are always options and it is, above all with prostate cancer, important to shape therapy to accommodate patients' needs.

Patient F was a 61-year-old accountant who was sent to me with a PSA of 98, confirmed on retesting. He felt very well and exhibited no symptoms. Work up showed that there was no evidence of bone metastases or lymph node enlargement. I explained that if he started hormones, this figure would come down and the prostate would shrink; if things went well perhaps in six months we could, along with my radiation oncologist colleague review whether radiotherapy would add to the possible control of the cancer. Well, he said, that was fine, but his wife who was a couple of years older, had become forgetful and had been diagnosed as early onset dementia. As her doctors could give him no prognosis, he felt he would go on to the hormones, have a follow up with me and see how things developed. As expected, his PSA fell to just under 2ng/ml, and remained like that for the next couple of years. His wife's condition only marginally deteriorated but was progressing in the wrong direction. As the PSA was steady, he agreed that only if it went up to over 10 should we restage him and see what further might need to be done. He felt the hormones had side effects he was unhappy with and had already had a couple of periods off when he felt better and more able to cope. As he was about to retire, he wished to formally enter an intermittent programme, having valued the 'off' periods. Our local protocol, at the time, used a value of 20ng/ml (to be discussed in detail later) as the value to trigger recommencement, and he was quite aware that eventually the PSA would not go down on recommencement. His own GP was happy to monitor this, and we parted, my expectation being that I would see him sooner rather than later. He didn't come back and I had taken semi-retirement when ten years later I bumped into him and his wife in the local supermarket. She was obviously more fragile, but he appeared no different. How was he? I asked. Just the same; he was off the hormones for six to eight months, and it was taking about nine months to get the PSA down when he started them again, but he felt much more active mentally and physically when not taking the drugs and was happy to soldier on. His wife's condition had worsened, but he felt fit and well to take care of most of the caring needs helped by family members; he did not wish to change the regime. I have no explanation except to say this was not the first time I had seen this durable response with hormones alone, and although studies in which I had participated showed no control or survival advantage to intermittent treatment, the reduction in side effects was very useful for this couple. He is now in his middle seventies, and many more options have opened up for him when this primary hormone therapy fails, if it ever will in him.

Whitmore first used brachytherapy ,the insertion of radioactive seeds into a tumour, via an open operation at the beginning of the 1970s.The disposal of the seeds was random, and the seeds themselves migrated, but the principle, used in other cancers such as tongue, appeared sound, and with the development of more sophisticated rectal ultrasound, it became possible to reconsider this as an alternative strategy. There was something of a misfire during the 1980s when the dose delivered was too high and rectal injuries were caused, but Blasko, in Seattle, refined the methodology and it was taken up by others. Initially, the cases chosen were low risk, and the prostate needed to be of a modest size, up to 50gms. They also tried to ensure no anatomical anomalies, and no adverse urinary symptoms. However, the method could be systematically delivered under a general or spinal anaesthetic, and it rapidly became possible to perform many cases in the day with the patient being discharged the same day.

Two types were initially used, low-dose rate (LDR) permanent seed brachytherapy where the 5mm seeds containing the radioactive isotope were permanently left in place, and this used iodine-125, caesium-131, or palladium-103. Iodine-125 became the most widely used.

The second which delivered a high-dose (HDR) brachytherapy, utilised a temporary implant or plastic catheters and Iridium-192 which delivered the dose in minutes and was then removed.

The low-dose system gained rapid acceptance, frequently patient led, and my colleague, Dan Ash, was the first to bring the technique to the UK in its current guise. The Leeds results, of 1,298 patients followed for 10 years are broadly representative of results elsewhere, but Blasko's results (2001) which brought this to prominence, in 125 patients, are worthy of quoting first. The biochemical relapse-free survival at 10 years for low risk was 87%, and intermediate risk 78%.

The Leeds group showed 89% for low,78% for intermediate, and 63% for high cases they took on as greater confidence was gained, and also represented some patients who had received an external beam boost if they had high-risk features.

The literature has numerous single centre reports of variants of these techniques.

There is, of course, never a free lunch, and this technique had both early or acute, and late complications.

Firstly, most patients had urinary symptoms of frequency, urgency, and mild pain or discomfort in passing urine. Around 10% went into acute retention of urine and required a catheter. If this was left for 10 – 14 days, most patients could void urine spontaneously on removal of the catheter. Some needed the catheter for longer, and a few required a surgical procedure, a bladder neck incision or channel TURP before they could pass urine.

Late effects included between 5 and 10% developing a urethra stric-ture which needed treatment. Urinary incontinence was rare and tended to be seen in patients who had had previous endoscopic prostate surgery. Impotence was still a problem at a reported rate of 15 – 40% of patients, but these figures tended to be consistently lower than for radical pro-statectomy.

As I visited the USA in the early years of this century I noted that the numbers of radical prostatectomies were in decline, from a high dur-ing the surge of 150,000 or more it had fallen to well under 100,000, and eventually seemed to settle at around 65,000 a year. I thought I was up to date with prostate cancer and its practice and knew of no new break-through in treatment for early stage prostate cancer; the incidence rate re-mained between 160,000 and 200,000 cases. Surely people were not choosing no treatment, and why were the urologists so sanguine as surely this, unlike our own system, would be affecting their income?

I need not have worried. The most skilled practitioners with TRUS were urologists, so most practices had hired a radiation oncologist to do the maths, and urologists delivered the therapy. Not inappropriate, as most of the complications were urological and needed to be sorted out by them. The number of cases rose to over a 100,000 a year; I believe com-pletely unsupported by any scientific evidence that it was equivalent to surgery, let alone superior. It was apparently patient led.

But the bottom line was probably the real bottom line for all 'stake-holders'. At this time a day care brachytherapy cost $9,000 whilst all surgery needed an overnight stay, even in the patient hotel, and couldn't be done cheaper than $12,000.

That the market is fickle and frequently devoid of logic we all know, and as we shall see, acts after its own fashion.

8. A Re-examination of Hormones

Although the Veterans' Studies appeared to have settled many questions with respect to hormone treatment, hormones work especially in advanced, symptomatic patients; early use in high-risk disease appears beneficial, the benefits are of variable duration, but all seem to fail eventually. The benefits of combining hormones with radiation therapy in locally advanced disease, and the fact that LHRH agonists had virtually taken over from orchidectomy as a treatment and some anti-androgens appeared very effective, but with a chance of preserving sexual function meant that many of these old questions were re-explored for the modern era.

A trial to see whether pre-treatment with hormones before radical prostatectomy showed no benefit from the hormones (Soloway 1995) but timing, and who should receive therapy was examined in some detail via RCTs as well as many cohort studies. A large MRC study from the UK compared immediate versus delayed which allowed both orchidectomy and LHRH agonists, showed that clinical progression in some patients was delayed but the mortality rate was not statistically different. In another large study by the EORTC, nearly 1,000 patients were randomised into immediate or deferred therapy. This was an older group of patients; the median age was 73. There was a modest overall survival advantage in the immediate group, but this did not come from controlling the prostate cancer, as prostate cancer mortality, and symptom-free survival were no different. This was a trial of great importance as it could not be replicated now. Patients on the deferred arm were not recommended to start hormones until they became symptomatic. Many, therefore, had lived with a rising PSA for some years, and a number had developed asymptomatic metastasis on bone scan before commencing their hormonal treatment. Despite this the most catastrophic disaster, paraplegia caused by bone erosion into the spine, only occurred in a handful of patients, slightly more in the immediate than the delayed arm, but obviously in view of the very small numbers, not significant.

What this did demonstrate was a confirmation of what was known – that hormones work in symptomatic patients. The median time for initiating treatment was 7 years, not dissimilar to the Hopkins figures following radical surgery. The patients lived a median of 5 more years, but more died from non-cancer causes, and in the delayed arm a significant proportion died before they had had to start hormone treatment (Studer 2008). A subgroup analysis did try to identify men with increased risk of death. Men whose PSA was greater than 50ng/ml, or had a PSA doubling time of less than 12 months, were more likely to die from prostate cancer, treatment immediate or delayed; those with values less than this were more likely to die from other causes.

These studies established a framework on which patient discussion about whether and when to intervene. There was no rush and patients could decide within this what they wished to do and whether other conditions they might have were a bigger threat to longevity. There is still a debate to be had. There was no survival benefit to early treatment, but patients often needed the psychological reassurance that 'something was being done'. As we will discuss later, the concept, in practice if not in name, of Active Surveillance had come to replace Watchful Waiting.

The side effects of hormone therapy are not trivial and these need to be considered very carefully in patients who may face many years on this therapy. Most earlier studies concentrated on the symptomatic or predictable side effects. Hot flushes (or flashes in North America), loss of libido, emotional instability, or fatigue, often quite profound. However, more recent work suggests that the morbidity (illness-inducing) effects of ADT are more insidious and lead to induction of metabolic syndrome leading to increased cardiovascular risk and the induction of osteoporosis and thus vulnerability to bone fracture. An observational population study in US Veterans (Keating 2010) in a cohort of 73,193 patients on ADT had a 44% increased risk of diabetes, and around 16% increased risk of cardiovascular disease including an 11% increased risk of sudden cardiac death.

Patient G was 74 and found to have locally advanced prostate cancer, declined radiation therapy after discussion but agreed to go on to a hormone study where he was randomised to immediate LHRH therapy with ten days of anti-androgen to cover the flare. He was fit, only on a single drug for hypertension (blood pressure) which was well controlled, and another for acid reflux. We ran a dedicated prostate cancer clinic, and initially gave the LHRH injection three monthly before this was carried out by his own doctor. We had a follow-up protocol because of his trial inclusion but usually three monthly. Over the first six to nine months he became withdrawn and fussy to a greatly exaggerated state. I was con-

cerned that he was depressed, which his family agreed to as he was be-coming very difficult to live with and putting a great burden on his wife. My psychiatric colleague felt he was not depressed and didn't need med-ication but he, like me, was convinced the hormones were directly re-sponsible for completely changing his personality. I suggested he come off medication, but he declined because he had cancer and needed the treatment. We and he were saved by the recently formed prostate cancer support group; when he went along to one of their meetings, he was bul-lied by another member to go to the gym. Once both his physical activity and socialisation were increased he began to become recognisable as his old self, and not as his daughter told me, at the same time telling me to sort it out (this is Yorkshire after all) an   old '-----'.

The next extensive studies of hormones followed the paper from Labrie in Canada, suggesting that if LHRH and an antiandrogen were combined, then the testosterone from the adrenal would be inhibited and a greater benefit would thus be obtained. This concept had been ad-dressed in the VACURG studied when orchidectomy and DES showed no better outcome than either alone. The initial findings, as they always do, showed very good results. A large number of RCTs were carried out to test this concept, by one estimate at least 27 with few able to replicate these good outcomes. A meta-analysis (a statistical manoeuvre that seeks to find common threads in numerous studies), most usually with different protocols, found that for studies in which 90% of patients had meta-stases, and had favourable prognostic factors, which usually meant that they started with only a small number of metastases, they were the only group to have increased survival at five years. When intermediate, and higher-risk groups were introduced, any benefit disappeared.

Patient H was a 62-year-old architect who presented with urinary symp-toms that required surgery. Physical examination and blood test showed no abnormality. He was one of three patients who had a TURP that morning, and all went well with them and they were discharged home after a couple of days. When I arrived to do a ward round a couple of days later, sister took me into her office. The pathology is back and all three of those from last week have got cancer; what are you going to do about it? Get them back next week and I'll talk to them and their relat-ives. Two of the three had incidentally found cancers: a small volume, less than 5% which I would not follow up, and was able positively to re-

assure them and their families. Patient H, however, had extensive Gleason 7 disease. I was flabbergasted; his prostate felt completely normal to me. I saw all of them, but the longest was with patient H. I explained that we needed to do a full cancer work up and then review what our options were. My distress worsened, for despite his PSA having risen a little, which I attributed to a post-operative effect, his bone scan came back positive, with numerous lesions. I was very tempted to get a bone biopsy as I didn't believe this could be so, but discussion with my radiological colleague convinced me it could be nothing else, and some x-rays I had done showed the characteristic dense lesions of secondary prostate cancer. He agreed to be randomised into a trial of combined therapy against LHRH alone and drew the combined therapy. His PSA, which had now risen into the low 20s, fell within three months to unmeasurable. He remained fit and well for seven years. No measurable PSA, and all the abnormalities in his bones disappeared. I thought I was seeing a genuine cure from hormones. Then, alas, the PSA began to creep up, and the bone lesions reappeared and became painful. He was treated with best supportive care, including going on to stilboestrol (DES)which brought the PSA down for a while, but he died just over two years after the rise in PSA, and I confess to being in denial that this could happen for longer than I should. Patient H benefited from the end of life care in a hospice, where he had worked as a volunteer when he was well and retained his concern for others to the end. I really thought, as had happened in other patients with other cancers, this time we had beaten the odds. He was only 71.

A further refinement of the use of hormones, and the first that showed the possible utility of LHRH agonists over orchidectomy, was the suggestion that intermittent hormone use could prolong the period for which the prostate cancer remained dependent on androgens. Behind this was the scientist Nick Bruchovsky, one of the discoverers of the androgen receptor (Akakura 1993). Put simply, the hope was that intermittent therapy would suppress activity but not kill off all the androgen-dependent tumour cells. When the androgen suppressor was withdrawn, sensitive cells would grow preferentially, and when the ADT was restarted these cells would be suppressed again, and so on and hopefully on. When you re-commenced the ADT was a matter of discussion, and I remember the EORTC, agonising over what would be safe as a PSA value before agreeing on 20ng/ml, this being the result everyone felt comfortable with. Our American colleagues arrived at 15ng/ml after the same tortuous talk. All of these were best guesses. The hypothesis had laboratory backing from the Canadian studies in the animal model of Shionogi mammary carcinoma, possibly a bit of a stretch.

My senior colleague and I had no doubt of its utility, however, and eagerly joined in the trials of this concept.

Patient I was found to have locally advanced prostate cancer aged 59. You can tell this goes back sometime, as he was on stilboestrol 1mg daily. We were very fortunate to have use of PSA in the early 1980s, as a monitoring blood test thanks to the late Professor Teddy Cooper, who was chair of Cancer Research, and a protein scientist, very interested in all sorts of tumour markers. When I reviewed Patient I, there was something odd about his results. For about six months in the year the PSA result was very low but for the other half it went up to the late teens before coming down again. He was being monitored three-monthly, as much to see how the marker worked as anything, and he had readily agreed to help us. I told him I couldn't explain the results, as elsewhere this marker had been pretty consistent in reflecting disease activity. Do you think staying on the tablets matters? he asked me. Certainly, I said. If you weren't taking them, then I'd expect the value to rise. Well, he said, you see, I run the funfair in the summer at one of the big parks in Leeds. I like to be on form, so to speak, during the summer, and these tablets do nothing for my prospects, so come April when I start back at the funfair, I stop them and start again in October when it closes. I really do like the nice warm feeling they give you, so that keeps me nicely during the winter. Internal water bottle as it were. I really don't want to stop the way I am taking them. And so he continued. A few years later he had a stroke and died but he had taught us that intermittent therapy was not dangerous and had positive advantages.

In a trial recruiting locally advanced and metastatic disease patients, more of the former than the latter, in 626 patients, there was no difference in overall survival, but a slightly increased risk of a cancer death (106 vs 84) which was balanced by a higher rate of death from cardiovascular disease (52 vs 41). A Southwest Oncology Group (SWOG) study was designed to specifically investigate the benefit in metastatic patients. It hoped to show that intermittent treatment was not inferior to Continuous Combined Androgen Blockade. In total 3,040 metastatic patients were recruited, and all commenced on CAB, but after seven months only 1,535 patients achieved a PSA less than 4.0ng/ml and could be randomised to either arm. The median and 10-year survival results were 5.8 years and 29% in the CAB arm and 5.1 and 23% in the intermittent arm. The most useful information to come from this study was provided by Hussain (2006). The response to PSA was the major predictor. Overall survival in patients whose PSA did not get below 4.0ng/ml was 13 months, 44months for those whose PSAs had got below 4.0ng/ml but remained above 0.2ng/ml, and in those where the value was 0.2ng/ml or less it was 75 months. Either approach would therefore seem reasonable in the right patient.

Patient J was a doctor who was the longest-lived male ever in his family at 57. There was a dreadful history of cardiovascular disease, taking the males in their late 40s or early 50s. He went into hospital under a neurosurgical colleague with debilitating back pain. An isolated abnormality in the first lumbar spine proved to be prostate cancer on pathological examination; biopsy of his prostate showed the same Gleason 8 tumour. Because of the ongoing pain which did not remit on starting hormones, he had a short burst of radiotherapy to the bone lesion and the pain fairly rapidly subsided. We had a discussion mostly about what he wanted to do. Well, firstly, he had planned to retire at 60 and still wanted to do that. He was sexually active and wanted a chance of preserving this, which he felt was important to his wife and him. He had plans for the first year after retirement but then would see how things fell out. We were looking at that time at sequencing hormones to try to gain time, as well as using intermittent therapy, so he was started on bicalutamide (see below). We used 20ng/ml as a cut off and would move to LHRH when the PSA failed to come down, and then stilboesterol. I felt that given the PSA response he had a good chance of 5 years symptom-free survival, but that the disease would eventually fail to respond, but new therapies might well be available. His first response was for three and a half years, then for twenty months, and then for fourteen months, but his bone scan went from the one lesion which always remained to multiple ones. He was tried on radioactive isotopes, which helped symptomatically, and then stopped any new medication and entered one of our hospices. It ran an outreach service that looked after him very well, and nine months after progression he died peacefully at home where he wished to be.

We found the use of intermittent therapy very helpful in younger patients, who felt more in control and findings that the survival of patients on bicalutamide was only six weeks shorter than LHRH pushed us to use it because of its lower side effects profile, and the possibility that sexual function could be preserved. We had tried sequencing (Kotwal, 2008), and showed that a series of responses could be obtained and following the scheme outlined for patient J. But, as expected, the first response was the best, and subsequently, fewer men responded, and those that did were for a shorter duration. Apart from best supportive care we had no ready new drugs to continue the sequence.

I was asked to see a patient with metastatic prostate cancer, Patient K, in one of the large prisons in our region. I had never met a murderer before and was asked to give a prognosis of his survival. There is nothing worse in medicine, as my friends and colleagues in Scotland found when faced with a much more criminally and politically charged case some time later. All of us have had patients who delighted in telling me that I had guessed at a year or so, and here they were five years later doing very well. Patient K's case appeared very tragic to me. He had been diagnosed with metastatic prostate cancer 3 years previously and commenced on hormones. Apparently, I have only his side of the story; his wife could not cope with his impotence, or possibly didn't understand it, but she had several flagrant affairs, and tormented him for his lack of erectile function. He flipped and strangled her, then gave himself up to the police immediately. Now it was thought he was dying and at present was in the prison hospital. Two of his children were still teenagers and were about to be orphaned. He was going into kidney failure, and although there were still some remedial measures that could be taken, he had refused all further treatment, and it was possible with his deteriorating kidney function to calculate how long he had, a couple of months at the best. That was my opinion. I have never had a sadder consultation and always wondered if matters between him and his wife could have been handled better. The side effects of hormones are a family problem, not just the patient's, and this reinforced my view that a clinic with time, and involving the whole family, however long that takes, must always be a necessary adjunct to managing all patients with prostate cancer.

9. New Technologies: I Robot

The role of laparoscopy, initially as a diagnostic tool using a camera inserted into the abdomen, filling the abdomen with air, and then carrying out an inspection (laparoscopy) of the abdominal contents had been used since the 1960s, frequently by gynaecologists to inspect the pelvis and its organs, but optics and instruments did not allow any more sophisticated manoeuvres. As optics, light sources and instruments improved, operations laparoscopically developed, the commonest early one being a cholecystectomy (gall bladder removal).

In 1997 Schuessler, a member of Ralph Clayman's group, performed the first laparoscopic radical prostatectomy, but it was the French, with tremendous Gallic verve, who took this technique and refined it. Abbou, Guillonneau and Guy Vallancien pushed these procedures towards being routine. The Montsouris technique was adopted and the outcomes in the short term, in relation to tumour clearance (margin positive rate), continence and retained potency in the early phase appeared similar to open radical prostatectomy.

The positive margin rate ranged from just under 10% in Jens-Uwe Stolzenburg's 2,000 cases (2008) to 15% in the Guillonneau series. Continence was between 83 and 92%, and potency in pre-existing potent men, where the nerves on both sides had been spared (as per the Walsh technique), was as high in one series as 100%, although this figure declined if ability to have intercourse was asked (65 -85%).

The patient was able to recover more quickly from this closed procedure, so that length of stay in hospital fell, and time taken to return to full normal activities was shorter. The downside was that the surgeon needed specific, spatial awareness, and whilst only a few lacked this facility entirely, the conversion time, or learning curve to achieve the same competence as open surgery, within an arbitrary time scale of four hours was long, and it appeared that at least 80 cases were needed to attain that proficiency. Surgeons already providing an excellent open radical prostatectomy service literally did not have the time to stop their practice with such a long and steep learning curve ahead of them. Providentially, the robot appeared.

The Da Vinci System was originally developed for cardiac surgery, but in 2000 Binder and Kramer performed the first robot-assisted laparoscopic radical prostatectomy (RALP). It is vital to note the 'assisted' surgery is not done by a robot, not yet anyway.

Although there are other systems, the Da Vinci is by far the most widely used, and almost all reported work has been carried out with this system. There are thought, currently, to be approaching 3,000 of these machines in use worldwide today (2018). It is described as a 'master-slave' system, which comprises a surgeon's console (master), a patient-side robotic cart (slave), and an image processing stack. The first generation of these systems had three robotic arms, two for instruments, and one for the telescope. The surgical field could be viewed, three dimensionally, in x10 magnification using stereo-endoscope and camera, and surgical instrument tips had a 360-degree range of movement. Newer models have introduced a fourth arm, and newer technology (EndoWrist) which provided even greater manoeuvrability for the surgeon. They operate the system from the console, looking at the console screen, but the deployment of the operating elements takes both a little time, and experience, and assistants are necessary.

The great attraction of this system was not just the chance for 'little boys and girls' to play with this wonderful machinery; although it was, in essence, only a laparoscopic prostatectomy, for the surgeon converting from open operations to laparoscopic ones, when one moved your arm to the right, that's what was happening in reality. The surgeon was able to convert to this system, if an expert prostatectomist very rapidly, some being back to their open best results within 10 or a dozen cases (Ahlering 2004). Reviewing conversions from open to laparoscopic, the robot-assisted appeared to need only 20 cases for a surgeon to become competent, whilst, as we have seen, 80 were required when the laparoscope was wielded by hand.

In 2002 Mani Menon and colleagues described the early outcomes from the technique, and the establishment of a structured program of learning the technique, and later the same year, Ash Tewari (2002) described how to carry out an anatomic radical prostatectomy, after Walsh, using the Da Vinci system.

A second, mini-surge ensued, and by 2008, an estimated 60% of the 65-70,000 radical prostatectomies were being carried out as robot-assisted laparoscopic procedures. It is estimated that by 2020 over 80% will be carried out by these means. Why?

Follow up in the majority of cases is still far short of the 15 years, at least, that will be necessary to assess equivalence to the open operation. The interim-reported outcomes are very favourable; no one ever publishes my 100 worst operations.

The positive margin rate, which in the reported series includes T2 (confined to the gland, clinically and by imaging), and T3 in which the capsule is breached, at least on imaging, has reported positive margins between 8.5% and 18%. Continence rates for large series, over 1,000, are over 90%, and when the patient had previous potency, the retained potency rate, if the nerves on both sides of the prostate were preserved, were also over 90%. Some meta-analysis has been carried out on this specifically and report a range of 63 – 100% if both nerves can be left intact.

These figures almost exactly replicate the excellent results from the 1980s after Walsh's new anatomical insights. The critical outcome is patient survival free from cancer, and what the prostate cancer-specific death rate will be at the critical 15 years' time of analysis; and this needs to be a real 15 years survived by all patients, not an actuarial projection. Nevertheless, not only are higher-risk patients being given the opportunity of surgery, the inevitable improvement in the technology should mean even better visualisation, and now a generation of surgeons trained completely, but only in this method.

This is not a cheap option for a struggling health system. And as we can see, its initial impetus was to allow patients to get the benefits of laparoscopic surgery, reduced blood loss, early discharge and more rapid return to normal activities. It appears a sensible investment decision, and the selling point of being operated on, in part at least, by a robot, was becomingly futuristic. It is difficult to arrive at meaningful costs in a multi-payer system, but costings in the single-payer system such as the UK, NHS, are measurable. The investment in the machinery itself is the biggest outlay, and in a capital-starved system such as the UK's, this expenditure is difficult to acquire, but where these are operating, and more are in place each month, an additional £1,200 pounds per case is added above the costs of an open radical prostatectomy. The more cases done, the lower the individual cost. We will discuss these ramifications later.

Finally, in the technology developments which assisted patients with problems post-prostatectomy came artificial urinary sphincters (AUS) and penile prostheses. Both of these were well developed by the mid-1990s and were available to men with intractable problems of continence or impotence. Both of these products were expensive in whichever system one sat and required surgeons of experience to obtain the best results. Nor were many patients following their operation suitable for anatomical reasons for even thinking that either might be a solution.

In a series of 40 patients, treated consecutively between 1997 and 2003, with the American Medical Systems 800 sphincter, 90% achieved continence, but even in expert hands the surgical revision rate, that is removal and replacement with a new one, was 20% at 10 years follow up.

A study by Chiang (2000) of 331 men who had penile prostheses inserted, showed a good overall outcome at 10 years, but 7% had needed the prosthesis changed because of mechanical failure, 6% removed because of infection, usually abscess formation, and nearly the same number because of either persistent pain, or penile swelling that did not resolve.

It is important to remember that these were just treatments for side effects and made no difference as to whether the operation had cured the cancer and only goes to re-emphasise that no operation is ever trivial.

10. New Drugs

New drugs began to come along, and these enlarged the current options. One of the first which did not directly impact on prostate cancer but on quality of life (QoL) was the licensing in April 1998, by the US FDA (Food & Drugs Administration) of sildenafil (viagra). One of the first studies (Zagaja 2000) looked at the effects of this agent on men post-prostatectomy who had been impotent for up to 18 months. In 170 patients there was an overall response rate of 29% but subgroup analysis looking at age and whether or not one or both nerve bundles had been preserved found that in the small group of men with both nerves intact, and under 55, 80% responded whilst no man over 55 with just one nerve bundle left intact responded. There was, as expected, no response in any group if both nerve bundles needed sacrificing.

A recent study (Jo, Jeong, Lee et al, 2018) looked at 120 patients who were classified as low on the International Erectile Function Index, and found that if treatment was commenced with PDES 5 inhibitors (viagra-like drugs), 41% achieved useful erections by the end of twelve months, but if started three months after recovery then only 17.7% achieved the same goal at a year.

A trial comparing functional outcomes between PDES 5 drugs (tadalafil in this case) and penile prostheses was carried out (Megas 2013) and using the International Index of Erectile Function where high is good, the prostheses scored 20.4 against the drug's 8.1. However, the questions posed were quite limited.

Because hormones had an almost miraculous outcome when used in patients who already had incurable, and often very symptomatic disease, when they failed most patients and doctors recognised that no patient would benefit from other than optimal end of life care. In 1981 a hybrid drug, estramustine (combining an oestrogen and a chemotherapy agent) was trialled and licensed for prostate cancer patients. There were some responses, but the toxicity was often such that few patients actually completed a prescribed course, and reinforced the view that chemotherapy had no place in prostate cancer treatment.

As more patients became into the category of castrate resistant, non-metastatic cancer attempts to use chemotherapy were persisted with, with greater keenness. In 1996 mitoxantrone, which had been used against a variety of tumours, was shown to have some effect on PSA, but in this particular group of patients the toxicity meant that few patients continued with the agent, and no complete disappearances, i.e. disappearance of all tumour, were reported. In 2004 Ian Tannock from Toronto led a study comparing docetaxel and prednisone, versus mitoxantrone and prednisone, and showed an advantage to the taxane drug. Subsequently, a large randomised Phase III trial (TAX 327) in 1,006 patients showed a clear, if small, increase in overall survival comparing these two regimes, of 18.9months, against 16.5months, and docetaxel became the first line therapy in castrate-resistant patients whether they had or did not have metastases.

Patient L had been diagnosed with locally advanced prostate cancer aged 68 and had entered a hormone trial where he received immediate therapy. He did well with a large reduction of his PSA from 62 to 1,3ng/ ml and sustained this position over several years. Six years from commencement his PSA began to rise, and a follow-up bone scan showed that he had developed three visible metastases, all within ribs. He, at the moment, had no symptoms from them. Taxane usage had just started and trials were still ongoing. My medical oncology colleague thought him suitable to treat off trial, and he commenced the drug. I had by now spent more than twenty years running this specialist prostate cancer clinic and chemotherapy had a very poor reputation with us locally. Patient K's daughter worked in our hospital and I bumped into her occasionally and always asked how he was doing. A bit tired, but none of the side effects they had been warned about. At six months, when he had long finished his course, and shown a gratifying drop in his PSA level, I saw him in our clinic. I told him of my scepticism, based on past experience, and asked what the whole experience had been like, as although fit at 74 it was not the ideal age to be tackling chemotherapy. Well, he said, he had been fine all through. He was very tired a couple of days immediately after the chemotherapy, but once this went, he was back to normal for the weeks before starting the next cycle. In his case the response lasted at least eighteen months, and he had a second response of a year before the disease remorselessly progressed and he died of prostate cancer in a hospice.

Unfortunately, only about half of the patients on taxanes respond, and many curtail their course because of side effects, not being so lucky as Patient K. The age group is not good for aggressive treatment, for as we will discuss later, even comparatively young men bring along a great deal of additional medical problems.

The taxanes were very useful, especially in the patients with no metastases who had ceased to respond to hormones; further trials found that another taxane, cabazitaxel, still gave responses following a full course of docetaxel, and gave useful responses in selected patients as second line treatment.

Rather like buses, you wait ages for one to come along, then suddenly four turn up all at once. It felt a little like this in the first decade of the new century. As well as real chemotherapy, at last having some effect in some patients, novel therapies were produced.

It had been most clinicians' experience that when the initial hormone began to fail in a proportion of men a second, and even a third response could be found, but these were with lesser numbers responding, and a shorter duration of response (Kotwal 2008). Nevertheless, there was a rationale for sequencing these agents, so that the suggestion that the cancer had lost all tumour responsiveness, at the first failure, was not true in everyone.

Over the last two decades, greater understanding about how the androgen receptor function occurred, and several mechanisms of how androgens could still operate were adduced. It was found that the enzyme (chemical messenger) CYP17 had an essential role in androgen biosynthesis. It was further noted that two drugs, ketoconazole and aminoglutethimide, which needed to be given with prednisone, were both non-specific inhibitors of the enzyme CYP17 and had modest effects in advanced prostate cancer patients, although many, because of the side effects, had reverted to only using steroids because of the side effects from these agents.

Abiraterone acetate was rationally designed at the Institute of Cancer Research in London, in collaboration with Cancer Research UK. Its action was as a selective inhibitor of CYP17A. It still needed to have steroids but in two Phase III trials, active agent plus steroids against steroids alone, in patients failing docetaxel treatment, there was a 4.6 months improvement in median overall survival. Nearly 800 men had received the drug, and its toxicity profile, even in this group of men who were a long way down the disease pathway in terms of pain and fatigue, was good, and this was accepted by most regulatory medicines bodies for use after first line chemotherapy. Instinctively, this felt to be the wrong place in the sequence, as was certainly the case with the next new arrival, enzalutamide.

In animal models the new agent, enzalutamide, showed activity when bicalutamide no longer evoked a response. Initial trials showed tumour responsiveness following docetaxel treatment, but there was concern that higher doses of the drug might be inducing seizures. However, a large Phase III study with 800 patients with hormone resistant metastatic prostate cancer, versus 399 patients on placebo, showed a median 4.8 month median improvement in overall survival, with an acceptable side effect profile, with the seizure rate minimal at 0.6%, although there were none in the smaller placebo arm.

Both these agents fit much more sensibly in a sequence before chemotherapy, and not unexpectedly new studies showed good and prolonged responses; the problems were as much getting the licence changed, despite the logic, as it was having to await the outcome of these trials. Neither of these agents were cheap but they did fulfil cost-effective criteria as laid down by some licensing and guideline organisations.

The concept of harnessing the body's natural defence mechanisms to combat cancer has always been logical but has proved to be very difficult in practical application. Some success has been met with the use of provenge (Eric Small 2006). This was a vaccine which was prepared using the patient's own cells, which in this case were dendritic (nerve cells) that needed to be harvested via a permanent long vascular line. A series of three treatments was delivered over a month and the patients so treated had several months of improved median survival. The cost, as will be appreciated, was far too high for routine use, but the scientific logic remains irrefutable; it's just not working in practice, yet.

Radioactive phosphorus was used to target bone cancers, both primary and secondary. The side effects were often lethal, and it remained, with respect to prostate cancer, a little-used agent. A safer, radioactive isotope, strontium 89, became available in the late 1970s and remained a workhorse of palliative care for prostate cancer patients with multiple tumours. It may have slowed down some, but it was its ability to stop pain and allow the patient to take minimal painkillers that made it so useful. It was combined with 'flash' radiotherapy for solitary areas of pain.

Patient M was a corporation road-sweeper. He presented with urinary difficulty, but the histology after a TURP showed Gleason 7 (3+4) prostate cancer, and on bone scan several metastases in his rib, hip and left humerus. He entered a hormone trial for metastatic disease and respon-

ded well. However, 20 months later, although his PSA was stable, in single figures, he came back complaining of severe pain in his left arm which was stopping him working. He went straight off for a single shot of x-rays, and over the week his pains disappeared. I talked to him about taking retirement due to ill- health, but he liked his job and wanted to continue as long as he could. Over the next three years, although his PSA climbed a little, the severe pain in his left arm lesion came back. The first time we did the same with the same gratifying result for many months before back he came again. I and my radiotherapist colleague were both getting worried, but he hadn't exceeded his permitted dose, the pain kept returning in the same place but always responded. This happened a total of five times, more than enough to allow him to retire when he wanted to, and start to have some form of leisure when he was admitted because of severe pain all over, and his bone scan had deteriorated, while his left, humeral lesion appeared as active as ever. This time he had strontium 89, which stopped all his pains, and he died a year later from a myocardial infarct, with no recurrence of any of his pains. Like so many of these cases I have no idea how or why he responded.

Radium-223 is the latest addition the array of isotopes available. Unlike strontium or samarium -153, which have not been shown to have any survival benefit but as we have seen a very good palliative effect, it has in trials shown a 3.6 month survival benefit, in metastatic disease, with a very low side effect incidence, although it appears it performs best when the patient does not have any secondaries elsewhere, only in bones – the majority of prostate cancer patients.

Bisphosphonates which have been extensively used in breast cancer have not proven so helpful with prostate cancer. One of the problems is that a whole new hierarchy of measurement, skeletal-related events (SREs) had been invented which showed that bisphosphonate delayed some of these, but as patients with prostate cancer were really only concerned with pain/no pain, and whether survival had been prolonged, which in the trial between the active agent and placebo it had not, taking yet more medication for no perceptible benefit was doubtful. Monoclonal antibodies have also been raised, but to date their benefit has not been obvious, another example where the logic of development is unarguable; it's just not working yet.

In the several thousand patients with prostate cancer who have been under my care, only one failed to show some response to hormones.

Patient N was 65 went admitted with acute retention of urine. Clinically his prostate was malignant, which proved to be so on histology. Bone scan showed multiple bony metastases, and he commenced on ADT. His PSA rose remorselessly; change of hormones, even several infusions of high dose oestrogens made not a scrap of difference. He was anaemic, had both low white cells and low platelets, so both isotope therapy and chemotherapy were precluded. We tried steroids; all to no avail. His disease took 10 months to kill him, the last few weeks being spent in one of our local hospices. I have never felt so helpless, but it remains unique in my clinical experience in not being able to do anything to halt, even temporarily, the march of this tumour.

And one has to accept that this is a cancer, and you can only do the best for the patient before you. One of the privileges of being a doctor is the chance to treat your colleagues and know they will return the favour. It can be both uplifting and a burden.

Patient O was a wonderful surgeon and a wonderful man. I'm sure that's the way round he would want it put. It literally took three people to replace him when he retired; and if your clinic in the old days had 100 patients, patient N's had 200, and he had hoovered up all the junior staff not doing anything specific to help. He fell suddenly ill whilst away lecturing, collapsed, was found to be profoundly anaemic, and was rapidly diagnosed with metastatic prostate cancer and offered an immediate orchidectomy, which he accepted. When he came home, we had a long talk. First it was obvious that he was unable to be a patient. We agreed that he would organise his own follow-up investigations and come and talk to me about them. I insisted that I see him with his wife, for I felt we had to be certain about time ranges and the inevitable outcome. I said that he probably would need supplemental hormone treatment, but he would be very unlucky not to get two years when he was pretty fit, although because all his presenting features were adverse, he could well need transfusions from time to time. Indeed he did, and arranged these himself. He wished to retire at 65, in a year's time. I thought that sensible, and our medical director, an old friend of us both, agreed as long as nothing untoward occurred to the patients. Patient O worked just as hard as ever for that year, had a great retirement do, many of the local surgeons having been trained by him, and continued to take holidays, being able to plan and devote individual time to each of his children.

He went to London to enrol in the new therapies which the Institute of Cancer Research were just bringing out into Phase II trials, but sadly did not respond. He was looked after by family and the hospice and its outreach service and died nine months into his third year from diagnosis.

Although I had exercised minimal control here, I felt, faced with the inevitable, we had managed to pause his disease, enable him to do what he wanted, offered hope of something new, which when it had failed, he accepted what was to come, and organised his end of life care. Nobody will emulate him, I'm sure, but I do feel, in prostate cancer, going on the patient's own terms is entirely feasible for virtually all.

The research activity of the last fifteen years has added further options to the sequencing of treatments available to patients with advanced stages pf prostate cancer. Recently two large RCTs, CHAARTED from the US, and STAMPEDE from the UK have further refined options. In both cases patients with metastatic disease not treated with hormones were randomised to either ADT alone or ADT with the addition of docetaxel and a clear benefit, in both studies, 56.6 vs 44 months. And 81 vs 71 months respectively, of the combination.

Thus, not only has creating a sequence now had a number of options, but high-risk patients, which they all were in these two studies, can have a more tailored regime.

11. New Imagining

The wide use of ultrasound scanning of the prostate (TRUS) and biopsy rapidly confirmed suspicions that the technique was probably erring in two directions. It was picking up a very large number of low grade, low volume lesions, but also missing significant disease.

Overdiagnosis was of greater concern as the diagnosis of a cancer inevitably led to treatment and its complications, when many of these lesions if left would never have created a problem in that particular patient's life. A study in the USA by Konety (2005) tried to replicate the autopsy studies of an earlier era. They could not find latent cancers which had been so ubiquitous in studies such as those of Franks. All the patients had had their PSAs done and their cancers diagnosed even if no active treatment had been rendered.

Significant disease, possibly in just the patients in whom surgery or radiation therapy might be curative, was being missed, primarily because in men presenting with a PSA of less than 10 the majority of tumours were not visible on ultrasound. Two strategies were adopted. Firstly, an attempt to make the ultrasound more sensitive by incorporating colour and power Doppler in highlighting vascular irregularities, and thus hopefully, focusing on possible tumours; and secondly on carrying out many more biopsies.

The numbers of biopsies rose from six to between 10 and 15 and then moved to the technique of saturation biopsies which incorporated 18 – 24 cores, which in some small prostates was actually carrying out a partial prostatectomy. This often needed to be done under a general anaesthetic and the increased yield appeared modest in comparison with the efforts that all, not least the patient, had expended.

Fortunately, the progress with technology allowed the MRI (Magnetic Resonance Imaging) scan to mature and multiparametric MRI emerged. This incorporates the opportunity to combine an anatomical and functional magnetic resonance sequence at a single examination.

There is a great deal of technological justification as to why this is altogether superior, but it may be summarised thus:

It appears to significantly reduce the number of overdiagnoses. When an MRI looks 'normal' it had tended to correlate with the absence of significant disease. In men who have had these scans and then gone on to radical prostatectomy, the pathology has correlated with significant disease forecasting, having a high detection rate of intermediate, and high-risk disease, Gleason 4+3, and Gleason 8 – 10. Paradoxically, it was more unreliable with low-risk Gleason 6 disease which is undoubtedly to the patient's advantage.

Greater use and greater knowledge will improve these factors, as certainly will new technological advances. And it is one of the areas where AI (Artificial Intelligence) looking at pattern recognition will come to play an increasing role. This is not to make radiologists redundant; an experienced group will always need to audit these outcomes and seek new developments.

The choline molecule is phosphorylated highly by malignant prostate cells and transported to the outer cell membrane. If it is attached with a radioactive label (C11 and F18 have both been used), then it has a sensitivity of detecting cancer cells. Sadly, there is quite a crossover in patients with BPH so it does not work well as a discriminant but is very useful in detecting lymph node disease. It is also less good at detecting sclerotic (dense) bone lesions which make up the majority of ones in prostate cancer, but much better with lytic (loss of bone) lesions such as can be found in breast cancer, for example. It is very expensive, and in practice is limited to those centres that have on-site cyclotrons to manufacture the tracer.

It is perhaps a short diversion to discuss briefly guidelines, as the introduction of np MRI has interesting lessons to be learnt. Guideline Committees in most parts of the world consist mostly of clinicians who review the current treatments, stage by stage for cancers, and increasingly for other conditions. Most review these fairly regularly, reflecting new research and reported outcomes of contemporary treatments, often every year or two. They therefore reflect current practice, but do not tell one whether it is correct or not. They do all have a hierarchy of evidence, from Level 1A, which is a meta-analysis of all RCTs on this particular subject, down through single randomised trials, cohort studies, the Level 4 which is expert opinion. Remarkably, many guidelines have no better evidence than Level 4. They should represent a dynamic view of best treatment options now, which will inevitably change, sooner or later. As an old boss of mine rather cynically put it, 'if you have a long enough period of reflection, you will find that the majority medical opinion at any one time will prove to be wrong,' but people, at any particular time, can only do what seems safest now.

The British National Institute of Clinical Excellence appears to have a somewhat different brief. It is looking for treatments that are under £30,000 per QALY (Quality Adjusted Life Year). This is a reasonable position; spending £300,000 on one patient to the detriment of many others is neither fair nor cost effective. This sometimes gets in the way of sense, however. Also, although clinicians are on the NICE panels and frequently chair them, the majority are 'stakeholders' who are non- clinicians. Their role except on cost looks disproportionate. The 2014 guidelines for prostate cancer failed to recommend npMRI for general NHS usage, although its results were already published and good, leaving UK patients to struggle on with TRUS whilst the rest of the high-income world had already transitioned to MRI usage. Because NICE does not review their guidance with anywhere near the frequency of all other guidelines bodies it will be several years before this anomaly is removed, leaving some hospitals in the UK able to provide this service while others cannot.

As will be discussed later, these are the sort of problems beyond the control of clinicians that could disadvantage their patients.

12. Active Surveillance, and the Search for Novel Therapies

Watchful Waiting was the most frequently carried out form of patient management in patients with prostate cancer, in the UK and Scandinavia, during the 1960s and 1970s, and formed the basis of the control arms for the handful of RCTs of radical prostatectomy. This was not nihilistic; radical surgery was not performed in these countries at this time, its poor reputation from the USA made few interested in taking it on. Most patients receiving active treatment had radiation therapy, and the results were mixed but compared well with the few surgical series, with on balance slightly fewer complications, although bowel disturbances were added to those of incontinence and impotence.

The rationale was that most patients were diagnosed over the age of 70 and had many co-morbidities which were likely to prove fatal long before the prostate cancer. The veterans' studies had persuaded most that early hormone treatment brought its own side effects, with little gain, as the treatment was palliative, not curative, except in patients with high-risk disease, a minority. Most patients, therefore, died with their prostate cancer, not from it, and unlike all cancers at this time, if patients did develop metastatic disease, hormones worked very well, adding at least two more good quality years to life. Many doctors who acquired the disease followed the logic and accepted, in the general scheme of things then, that it was one of the 'better' tumours to have.

The PSA revolution changed everything, as we have seen, and the over-expectation of cure by surgery led to many cases with a rising PSA, early treatment, and then castration-resistant non-metastatic prostate cancer, which in the mid-1990s had no ready, further treatment. It was also obvious to many that overdiagnosis was leading to overtreatment, with a deleterious effect on many (Whelan 1997).

Laurence Klotz, an academic urologist from Toronto, who had spent part of his training at Memorial Sloan Kettering in New York with Whitmore, put his head above the parapet and in 1996 proposed a different type of masterly inactivity, Active Surveillance. His initial target population were the large numbers of men with low-risk cancers, locally confined (Tic, T2a), Gleason 6 or less, and presenting a PSA of less than 10. It is difficult, at the height of the surge, to indicate the courage this took.

Patients were naturally anxious, and Klotz and his colleagues built in many tripwires to steer patients back towards interventionary treatments.

First, patients needed regular PSA testing, eventually settling at three-monthly for two years, and six-monthly thereafter. He also arranged that the initial group would be further biopsied at two, five, and then ten years, and irrespective of biopsies; if PSA doubling time was less than three years, these patients were referred for definitive therapy. In his initial reported group of just under 300 patients ,the median doubling time was 7 years, with 42% of the group being more than 10 years, and by extrapolation, 20% would need 100 years for the PSA to double, a problem none of them would have.

In the febrile atmosphere into which this was introduced the multiple testing was obviously very necessary. There was already enough information to be confident that radical surgery at least could be deferred for many months, mostly drawn from major centres' experience in the 1980s, when waiting times to have an operation at one of these were often measured in months, and the patients were correctly informed at the time that this delay did not make any difference to outcome.

As more data has been accumulated from Klotz and others this approach has gained wider acceptance; a UK survey by McVey (2010) showed 39% of patients had accepted this method of initial management, and a review by Holmstrom from Sweden, also in 2010, showed that outcomes in these patients, whether immediate or delayed (the average was 19 months), made no difference to the outcomes. Allied to this, early results from the PIVOT and Scandi4 radical prostatectomy studies were not demonstrating a huge difference in outcome for the surgical arm over the no therapy ones.

Although rational, and possibly overprotective, these results have not readily translated into popular understanding as a small survey study in 2012 (Xu 2012) demonstrates.

He carried out in-depth interviews in 21 patients (14 blacks,7 whites) who were newly diagnosed with localised prostate cancer. 14 of these had low-risk disease. As part of this survey, the option of Active Surveillance was asked about, as to knowledge, and to acceptance as a form of management. 19/21 opted for active therapy, either surgery or radiation therapy, one took a novel treatment, cryotherapy (see later), and two only enrolled on an Active Surveillance programme similar to that suggested by Klotz. One university professor in the group had consulted no fewer than eight physicians before opting for treatment.

Although this is a small study, one I carried out with the help of Prostate Cancer UK records very similar opinions.

Most having had a diagnosis just 'wanted to get rid of it or be cured'. Few had information concerning AS, and when told about it considered it to equate to 'doing nothing'. Some who did consider it were persuaded by family, friends and their physicians to think about active treatment. Many felt that they found it very difficult to reconcile the messages they had received, starting in the 1970s and the 'War on Cancer', and the continuing claims that 'early diagnosis and early treatment saves lives' with this proposition. Even though they felt they had been fully counselled as to the significant side effects of treatment, the majority felt that this was the only way to go.

Patient P was a senior civil servant diagnosed with prostate cancer while working in Europe. He consulted me, amongst many, as to his possible course of action. His work up, which was very comprehensive − this was a very well-respected major centre − showed he fell into the low-risk category, which I recommended would be suitable for an Active Surveillance programme after Klotz's schema, as he was just 59. He obviously received other advice concerning surgery radiation therapy which included brachytherapy, which felt him not a good candidate because of his urinary symptoms. He was strongly recommended to have surgery in Europe.

I tried hard to persuade him, something I rarely do because I felt he should get his urinary symptoms sorted out, and he could always opt for active treatment when he was ready if he wished. Both his physician adviser, but also his family, especially his children, advised him to go ahead with surgery, which he duly did. He had a horrific time with lack of urinary control which took us a few months to correct and stabilise, but since his operation, more than ten years ago, his PSA had been undetectable, with medication his urinary symptoms are controlled, but only one nerve could be spared, so that impotence has been the outcome. This patient, I believe, represents many of the dilemmas of a patient faced with the choice of Active Surveillance. The messages in the UK and Europe have been no different to those in the USA. The patients can often feel guilty that they are not doing everything and are somehow letting down their wives and children. Only more information can redress the balance between a chronological life possibly saved and an active life lost.

The problems of all observational or deferred treatment are what triggers make the doctor advise the patient to move to an active treatment choice and will that treatment be as successful as if the patient had decided to have it straight away. There is no evidence that delay is detrimental, but in the occasional patient this could happen, and we have no predictors to help identify who this could be. It will be recalled that the use of 15 or 20 ng/ml PSA value, which has been used for intermittent therapy, was chosen in a very arbitrary fashion; the level when all clinicians still felt the patient was safe.

A more scientific level was proposed by Richard Sylvester and Laurence Collette, statisticians of the EORTC group on that organisation's study of immediate versus deferred hormones in patients with initial localised or limited locally advanced disease, in which virtually all the patients from both arms had been followed until death. They found on analysis that only those patients whose PSA rose above 50ng/ml predictably and universally developed metastases. This important observation from a RCT followed to its logical endpoint means that we can expand the level at which hormonal treatment has to start, as no evidence exists to show starting it sooner gives the patient any advantage, but could also raise the level for recommencing hormones in intermittent therapy, and possibly a useful level in patients choosing radiation therapy, but it is difficult, in the present climate of belief, to see surgical treatment being withheld while the PSA climbed into the 20s or 30s, even though, at present, this is an evidence-free area.

How high can a PSA go before treatment is essential? I, like everyone else, have no idea, but probably a great deal higher than most people think.

Patient Q was a recently retired academic, aged 66. He was very fit and on no medication. He had had a check-up with his own doctor as he was about to embark on an extensive climbing expedition, which was his passion. A PSA had been done which came back at 416ng/ml. A repeat had pushed it up to 419ng/ml. I saw him a couple of days after the second result. I explained that I could not believe he did not have metastases, even if he had no symptoms. These, I felt sure, would come sooner rather than later, and would require treatment. To make him feel better I sug-

gested he start treatment straight away even before we had his scan res-
ults in.

Well, he said, he was off to climb several peaks in the Caucasus, in-
cluding the highest one, Mount Elbrus. All the arrangements had been
made, he felt very well, and looked up the side effects of hormones, as he
thought I might want him to go on them, but really, he'd rather not. He
didn't want weakness or fatigue during this trip. So, what was the worst
that could happen? I said he had a 1% chance of becoming paraplegic,
which would be permanent, and given where he wanted to go, probably
kill him. He had a very high chance of getting bone pain, which often
didn't respond to opiates, and he could become profoundly anaemic, and
that would probably kill him too. And what's the really bad news? he
then asked. So, off he went, and we agreed on his return he would repeat
his blood test, let my secretary know he was back, and she would book
him an urgent bone scan. About four months later he reappeared in my
clinic. I knew he was back, as he had carefully arranged his bone scan
as soon as he touched UK soil. His PSA was now 960ng/ml. But the bone
scan showed only a couple of probable metastases in his ribs, which he
said were not painful. I persuaded him to commence hormones, because
even if his sang-froid enabled him to view the progress of his cancer
with equanimity, I couldn't cope with a patient whose PSA was about to
go over a thousand without him receiving treatment.

Despite the incredibly high PSA, he did respond to treatment but
did die of his prostate cancer some four years later. Whenever we met,
he always thanked me for letting him climb his mountains. I continued to
acknowledge ruefully that that was the opposite of what I had planned
for him.

Active Surveillance has been shown to be safe for the majority of
patients, and when delayed active treatment has been instituted, to date,
the patient has not suffered detrimentally from not having immediate
treatment. It is a very viable option.

New treatments for localised Prostate Cancer

The obvious continuing existence of significant side effects from the major therapeutic modalities of surgery and radiation therapy meant that a
search for an effective, locally delivered therapy, which had a better
chance of preserving continence and potency whilst still controlling or
eliminating the tumour, was a natural direction to search. Several modal-

ities have been explored over the last two decades; one, cryotherapy, has had formal approval in several countries, two others have conducted Phase III trials, HIFU and PDT, whilst there is Phase II data on two other systems, IRE and Photothermal.

As can be seen, most of these must be seen in the context of experimental therapies and should only be given in units in experienced units whose outcomes are closely monitored and regularly reported.

Cryotherapy had a brief outing in urological practice as a possible method to treat benignly enlarged glands in the 1960s, but the complication rates were so high it was swiftly abandoned. Its return reflected the advance of technology in better imaging, and smaller probes which could deliver a more controlled 'ice ball' in the prostate, and thus destroy tissue.

The method was initially used in patients where radiation therapy had failed to destroy the tumour, and later treatments of newly diagnosed cancers were used. This treatment can be delivered as a day case, and the reported results have been variable; positive biopsies after treatment being between 4 and 45.5%, erectile dysfunction, 14 – 42%, and incontinence, 0 – 4%. Like any new therapy, limited in distribution, the more experienced units tend to have the better results. As we have discussed elsewhere, therapies that work and need to be delivered to hundreds of thousands of patients each year, worldwide, need to have a consistent delivery with a very narrow range of outcomes and complications. Whatever its other problems, surgery and radiation therapy has achieved this.

HIFU (High Intensity Focused Ultrasound) is a thermal energy technique that destroys cancer cells by heating, with the temperature rising to 56 degrees C in the target whilst sparing intervening tissue. It too has been employed in both salvage and primary treatments, and its early prototypes have been in action since 1993. Phase III trials have reported the following outcomes: positive biopsy, 8 – 23.5%, erectile dysfunction, 5 – 46%, incontinence, 0 – 5%. The technology here continues to advance.

IRE (irreversible electroporation), as the name suggests, uses electrical current to cause tiny breaks in the individual cell membrane which then leads to cell death. This is still at the early stages of developments, but Phase II trials have shown that it has some effect, and worthy of further study.

PDT (photodynamic therapy) is based on the activation of a photo-sensitiser by light on a given wavelength. Similar techniques have been used in the treatment of benign prostate disease, and superficial or non-invasive bladder cancer. It has, probably, currently made the most progress and should have Phase III trial results, comparing it against surgery in due course.

All have shown some usefulness, but none has yet to show consistent outcomes with minimal complications, although the goal of trying for therapies that do not replicate the complications of surgery and radiation therapy whilst maintaining its own modest long-term gains must, surely, be encouraged.

13. What is to be done?

Objectively speaking, we have not progressed a great deal further in our understanding, and therefore, treatment of prostate cancer in the last forty years, despite superficial signs to the contrary.

The small group identified by Walsh and Jewett that might be cured by surgery has had some support from the Scand4 trial ,which showed an absolute benefit of 11% for surgery over Watchful Waiting to be followed with ADT on progression, which means that seven patients will have had the operation unnecessarily for one to benefit. The longitudinal PIVOT study was even less helpful showing only a 3.5% difference in prostate cancer death rates in favour of surgery, well over twenty patients having to have surgery to benefit on their figures.

The ProTech study has as yet only got 10-year data, but what this had told us so far is confirmation that prostate cancer is a slow disease because at 10 years, out of nearly 1,700 patients, only 17 had died, 8 in the Active Surveillance arm, and 9 in the intervention arms, 4 with surgery, and 5 with radiation therapy. Only at 15 years follow up will we get any indication whether interventions have reduced the rate of disease progression, and probably only at 20 years will we be able to see if a significant difference in the death rate has occurred and been maintained.

A lot of men will be diagnosed with prostate cancer before these results are published, so this aspect of diagnosis and what to do needs addressing now.

ADT, as Huggins showed, and as the Veterans' Trials of the 1960s and early 1970s showed, works, and at any stage, imposes a rolling back of the disease for a period of time. We have surely proven conclusively, by inventing a new disease, non-metastatic castrate–resistant prostate cancer, by treating numbers, not patients, that hormone therapies work best for widespread disease, and now that we do have other agents that show some responses in prostate cancer, albeit not the near-universal and almost magical effects of ADT, this should be reserved for later in the disease.

How can we synthesise all the information we have and consider a regime that is safe for the patient but enables them to function for as long as possible normally, which is normal for them?

First, we must reinforce some old myths from previous eras: this is still prostate cancer, and whatever the claims, nearly 30,000 Americans continue to have their deaths attributed to this cause, just as was happening forty years ago. However much wriggling goes on, an attempt of mass eradication of prostate cancer of whatever type, maximally over twenty years ago, and therefore plenty long enough for a mass effect to be seen, has not shifted this figure, and the argument that the number of men from the 'baby boomers generation' means that the death rate has fallen, is at the margin at best, just as the 4% rise in deaths from prostate cancer reported this year (2018) is also only likely to be variation around a constant number. When interventions work, such as for cardiovascular disease in men, death rates fall by a half; where effective screening is allied to early treatment, such as with cervical cancer, the death rate plummets by two-thirds. We have to recognise that we are not seeing this with prostate cancer; indeed, in the UK, from the 8,000 deaths from prostate cancer in 1980, more than 10,000 are now recorded. Some of this must be larger numbers of men at risk, but even if that is accepted, and I will have something further to say about the UK's unique organisational response to these clinical outcomes, despite several thousand surgical operations being performed in the UK each year for the last 25 years at least, it is obvious that we are not going anywhere either.

Second, as the small study by Xu showed, because all cancers have been swept up in one mass, mass solutions have been offered which may not be appropriate, and indeed, possibly detrimental to patient outcomes. The War on Cancer, which commenced during the Nixon administration, by calling up the image of conflict, forced particular stereotypes on cancer sufferers. Not fighting the cancer, or if the disease gained, not fighting hard enough, unconsciously placed an immense and extra burden on patients already facing what was going to be a lethal disease, whatever their personal attitude to it. The misnomer arose because there had been a genuine effort to massively increase the money available for care and research, and the closest analogy was the mobilisation of resources for war in which the USA's contribution had been prodigious. This was similar, and quite a number of clinical and pure research organisations around the world benefitted from the American largesse. The EORTC, of which I was an active member, received US subsidies right up until the early 1980s. The myth, however, of a war in which the individual patient was a combatant, and the outcome of their 'fight' with cancer was determined as much by their moral attitude, as it was by the aggressiveness of the tumour itself, was unfair and tended to place the patient, already having to cope with a life-altering diagnosis, also somehow to blame as to whether they did well or not from the treatment of their tumour. It is no one's fault, least of all the patient with prostate cancer.

Early diagnosis and early treatment equate to cure. Most people agree that surgical treatment of early prostate cancer is curative (the word 'potentially' having long past slipped from the description). This is factually true, in that most people do agree; it is also wrong. A small group at best, those with localised disease and favourable prognostic factors, almost certainly the same group that Walsh identified, may be cured by early surgical intervention, but we are still a long way from knowing what these factors are which enable this to happen. This presumes that the Scand4 trial is true, and this has been dismissed as not relating to contemporary practice. Only when contemporary practice puts up proper twenty-year follow up in a randomised trial, not retrospective cohort reports, will we know whether contemporary practice is even as good as this, or whether the PIVOT study is actually indicative of surgical outcomes long term.

Let us therefore look how a more individualised treatment regime can be constructed and look for the upsides and downsides of any decision that a patient is faced with, and trust that it is not like some clinics in the UK which sent patients away with three leaflets, one each for surgery, radiation therapy and active surveillance, and asked to come back the following week and let them know which option they had chosen.

Unequivocally, this is a slow disease, and often a very slow disease. There is a great difference in rapidly arriving at a diagnosis which everyone one would like. This is not subject to targets but today, although yesterday would have been better. There are, in any system, time-limited stages. All of these should be as short as possible, and as happens in many places in high-income countries, all data can be available within a week. I always tell patients that this is the situation, i.e. the extent of their tumour should the diagnosis be positive, that there are a number of options, whatever state or stage they are at, and then to advise them to take a short break, as this will have been a distressing time for everyone involved with them, and they deserve a pause. Absolutely nothing is going to happen to them from the prostate cancer perspective.

As 90% of diagnoses are of men with localised disease, this needs to be considered first. I think it helpful to categorise men into the under 60s, which represent no more than 10% of the prostate cancer population, but they are in a group that does merit even more tailored discussion than the next group, 61 – 70, 71 – 85 and the over 85s. You will have seen already that many reports have different cohorts, e.g. 55 -64, or 65 – 74, etc., making comparisons difficult. What we have to understand about all patients is how fit they are and what their life expectancy is given that only 1% of patients are likely to die of the cancer in the first 10 years, whatever we do or don't do. I know that this is only definite for low- and probably intermittent-risk patients, but these are the vast majority, with again perhaps 10% falling into the high-risk category.

Ten years is often the benchmark quoted as far back as the 1970s for or against active interventions, but how accurate these predictions are is vitally important. A life table shows the probabilities of a member of a particular population living or dying at a particular age, and from this the remaining life expectancy for people at different ages is derived. When life table predictions were set against actual observed life expectancy, the tables overestimated the predicted life expectancy by 97% vs 81% for the observed. Although life tables try to make adjustments, they only average the co-morbidities, so must be inaccurate, to some extent when looking at the individual. The Charlson co-morbidity index tried to get around this problem, and life expectancy tables showed a predictably worse overestimate in patients with higher Charlson scores, but even with patients with low Charlson scores, the overestimate was still substantial.

In a retrospective, large cohort study of American patients (Daskivich, 2011), with non-metastatic prostate cancer, predominantly low- and intermediate-risk patients, with a median follow up of 6 years and an overall prostate cancer mortality of 3%, patients with Charlson scores of 0, 1, 2 and 3+ had a non-cancer mortality of 17%, 34%, 52% and 74% respectively. These, like many such studies generate a hypothesis, but a RCT is necessary to get nearer the truth. It has been found that an independent opinion on co-morbidities which is more accurate than life tables, can be obtained from a physician, not a urologist or an anaesthetist 'having a go'. Why this becomes of increasing importance is because recent figures have shown in men that whilst their life expectancy, as a function of time, has increased by 10 years since the Millennium, the wellness of this population, i.e. those not on medication of some sort, has only improved eighteen months, from about 62 to 63 and a half. Part of any discussion of prostate cancer therapies must first demonstrate to the patient that if he falls into the small group who predictably will benefit from intervention, he will be around to reap that benefit.

A couple of other points need establishing before discussing how different groups might be offered options with the primary purpose of maintaining good functioning health while at the same time minimising the risk from prostate cancer. The myth aimed at here is again that urgent action needs taking; it does not. No one ever died from a prostate cancer that stayed within the prostate. All interventional therapies have as their justification, cure, and when this doesn't happen, then the possibility of disease spread has been minimised. No retrospective or prospective cohort studies can give clear answers here unless virtually everyone had a favourable outcome; this happens if low-risk patients are treated, but this is exactly the same group in which demonstrably patients die with, not from their prostate cancer. The belief that early detection must pick up disease, which will turn into high risk if left, can on the evidence we currently have only be applied to a small number of patients, 10 – 12% at best, and we still have not been able to identify these individuals. We have had a twenty-year period of 'slash and burn' but the same numbers (actual not actuarial) of men continue to die from the disease. In high-risk patients, or those that turn out to be such and are not helped by interventions, rather like Elvis, the tumour may already have left the building.

The second point, which cannot be emphasised often enough, is that the worldwide introduction of PSA has moved back the diagnosis by ten years. This is why even fifteen-year follow-up data in the modern era is too little and twenty- to twenty-five-year material is needed to get an accurate idea of what is the natural history of this disease, untreated and treated. The Protech trial with only 17 patients dying of prostate cancer, actually, in the first ten years of follow up, reinforces the message of slowness of growth and time to think in many tumours.

Given that most patients being diagnosed are in the last quarter of their lives, the focus must surely be to preserve all functions for as long as possible, compatible with patient safety from the prostate cancer spreading. Many patients will not live to see the benefits of treatment or the consequences of misjudgement, but all treated patients will instantly develop side effects, with which many will have to live to the end of their days; npMRI might just be the new imaging modality that enables a safe path to be constructed for most patients.

Two small but very important groups need to be looked at first before the bulk of the patients are considered.

About 10%, or probably less of all cases of prostate cancer are diagnosed in men who are under 60. Exceptional cases can be found under 50 but each will constitute, even more than most, a unique therapeutic dilemma. Forty years ago, it was thought that getting prostate cancer young meant that the cancer was peculiarly aggressive because the observed survival of these patients anecdotally appeared shorter than their elder victims. However, analysis, stage for stage, showed that the survivals were the same, only ten years in a fifty-something, was still a premature death. The ten year benefit of PSA usage needs to be added, but we are still faced with the problem that it is likely that only a small number of men will get a cure that prevents them dying of prostate cancer, whilst many others will get only complications from treatment, and many would never have needed intervention anyway. Looking thirty years ahead, especially in a fit man on no medications, is a difficult projection.

They must be told that there are several months to discuss this problem before a decision is made. By default, they should go on a surveillance regime, with three-monthly PSA testing, and a repeat of their imaging when they have decided. It takes a great deal to cope with having a cancer and not doing something about it. Internal pressures within oneself, concern that you are not doing the best for the family is very difficult, and requires patience, often the help of other professionals to help the whole family, and a realistic anticipation of the side effects must be made. When the prospect of sexual dysfunction is raised frequently, in my experience, the wife or partner will say quite adamantly, that this loss doesn't matter, as long as he is all right. They do need to know that he will be all right for many years, and that late intervention does not appear disadvantageous, as long as careful monitoring is conducted.

As a guide for all prostate cancer patients, a number of risk tables have been developed. The first in the field was Alan Partin's, based on the Hopkins data. From this came the groupings of high, intermediate, and low risk. Other categories, ultra-low risk, for example, have followed. These are broad brush, and the outcome data from one specialised centre whose figures are likely to be in the top 5%, rather than representing the average. Nevertheless, they can prove helpful to the patient.

Low risk incorporates a PSA less than 10, a Gleason grade less than 7 (which in the current era will be 6, as grade inflation has removed the lesser ones), and a clinical stage (or more usually imaging stage) T1/2a, the old stages A and B1.

Intermediate incorporates a PSA less than 20, a Gleason grade of 7, and clinical stage T1/2b.

A high risk incorporates a PSA higher than 20, a Gleason grade 8 - 10, and a clinical stage T2/3a.

Many subgrades can be created, but prognosis in terms of biochemical rise free, overall survival, and prostate cancer-specific survival, broadly follow these paths, so that a high PSA even with everything else favourable will do less well; similarly, a higher clinical stage, or a higher Gleason score, will all tend towards a worse prognosis, even in isolation.

So here we have the young man's agonising choice: even if most things are favourable, there is apparently still a group whose tumour nature could change, and therefore he would benefit from surgery or radiation therapy. Active Surveillance with a move to active intervention if any parameters on the blood test or the scans should, currently, be safe and allow many younger men to avoid complications for a long period of time. But can a patient feel really well with a sword of Damocles hanging over his head? Some can and some cannot. There is not a wrong answer in this situation, merely trying to shape the treatment to the individual. It is disingenuous to tell the patient that the operation, radiation treatment will cure him, because nobody knows; but if the patient has had time and space to weigh up his options and what he wishes to do and decides he wants 'rid of it', then that is what will undoubtedly be what does best for that individual. A phlegmatic person with a great deal more to do than worry about his prostate will do equally well on a surveillance regime. Research, meanwhile, needs continuing focus on what it is in the blood or the tumour of an individual to sit passively in one and be life threatening in another.

The second special group is again about 10 – 12% of patients: those with high-risk disease, which will involve a high PSA, a Gleason score that is 8 or greater, and abnormalities on scanning showing the possibility of local extension beyond the prostate's edge, or any or all combinations. Until comparatively recently, Jewett's findings that none of these patients benefited from surgery have remained in the urological community's mind. Of the several thousand patients undergoing radical prostatectomy at Johns Hopkins by Walsh between 1992 and 2008, only 175 patients at high risk were found and separately analysed, these not being found until the final pathology report was through. Unfortunately, actuarial figures, not actual ones, were given as 10-year values, but two- thirds had remained free from biochemical progression, and thus the need to start any additional therapy. Similar, but more reflective of average practice, I feel is the study from South Carolina, where between 1987 and 2008 (again we are into actuarial, not actual territory), mean follow up was 53 months and median 49 months, from 3,755 patients who had surgery; 358 had Gleason number 8 or greater, so while the whole group produced about a two-thirds freedom from biochemical progression, if the groups were subdivided further, a group with everything adverse, only 26% escaped biochemical progression, which is what one would anticipate and all patients would need fifteen-year follow up to even begin to make any sense of this. Nevertheless, in recent years surgery has been offered to younger men with high-risk features, with a reasonable chance that some benefit will accrue, if only in delaying the disease, but as always the follow up is too short; proper trials could have been conducted as this was known to be a problem more than thirty years ago, so that making this choice is more like choices patients are faced with in other cancer types, and is an addition to the radiation therapy which for thirty years has been the mainstay of treatment in these high-risk patients.

In the absence of proper trials it is difficult to advise the patient whether or not there is the 'right' moment for treatment, and delay would lose the patient the opportunity for cure, but sufficient information is available in these patients that confirm the slowness of progress, and that PSA numbers can safely rise into the twenties or even thirties, to mean that Active Surveillance, at least initially, is not a dangerous option. Time can be taken to think this through and arrive at an individualised answer.

Trials of adjuvant (additional treatment) using early radiation treatment if cancer is thought to have been left behind appear no better than giving the radiation therapy later, and there are significantly fewer side effects from the added therapy if it is delayed. Giving hormones with or immediately after surgery does not help, whilst it, as a short course, does help the radiation therapy. The nerve bundles are more likely to need to be sacrificed in these cases so that restoration of potency is inherently more difficult, and patients going forward for this treatment probably need to accept that this will be the consequence of the treatment.

The majority of patients fall into the low- and intermediate-risk categories, and from 60 onwards will be the ones in whom increasingly other diseases will determine their life chances. Preserving continence and potency into someone's 70s is a very important quality of life feature. Recent surveys suggest that sexual enjoyment for both sexes is maximal in their mid-sixties, although other diseases and medications may impact on this. Understanding the length of time of this disease, and knowing what a patient's time might be, is massively important in allowing them to come to decisions that suit the individual. As a crude rule of thumb, you are much more likely to be fit and well in the next five years than the following five years, and so on. Of course, there will be exceptions, but a default position of active surveillance should be general for this large group. They have time to change their minds, many years of time.

The action by American patients to vote with their feet for brachytherapy, in the complete absence of evidence, may well be driven by economic factors, but a lot must be because of the presumed minimising of side effects while apparently achieving the same outcomes. Although progress seems slow at present, the quest for other forms of therapy is sensible but it still speaks to what is an outmoded narrative in prostate cancer that early treatment cures, and the earlier the cases are found, the better.

In October 2011 the United States Preventive Services Task Force (USPSTF) gave PSA-based screening a D recommendation, which suggested that PSA testing not be pursued as there was a 'moderate to high certainty' that the service had no benefit, or that the harms outweighed the benefits. Since then there has been constant lobbying by various interest groups, some exercised by the apparent rise in the last few years of the prostate cancer death rate by 4%. It will be apparent that a rise now in deaths reflects what happened 15 or more years ago, and the underlying actual statistic is that the US number of deaths attributed to prostate cancer remained around 30,000 a year, exactly where we were in 1980. Nevertheless, the USPSTF issued new guidance in May 2018, moving their recommendation to a C, which suggests men should discuss the value of having the test performed with their physician, and accept the known risks of overdiagnosis and likely overtreatment unless active surveillance is where most of them start.

It has become fashionable to use PROMS (Patient Reported Outcomes), the same method used by Fowler and colleagues among US Veterans in 1990 -1994, with alarming reports, as we have seen, because everyone thought that surgical outcomes everywhere would replicate the Hopkins, St. Louis or Mayo figures. The current concern is found consistently in prostate cancer patients who have had interventions, experienced side effects in the first year predictably from continence and erectile dysfunction; when asked at the end of year 2 about their general wellbeing, it is frequently positive even if some side effects appear now to be long standing. The cynic would suggest, if the patient felt that without treatment he would, like other cancer patients − lung, pancreas, for example − be dead in a year; even if he wasn't told this no one knows what goes on in people's minds: being alive and really quite well two years down the line must give anyone a psychological boost.

It is what patients generally must understand − the reality that the huge period of time the disease gives them, and by going into active surveillance, it signals to the patients that this is a slow tumour, and no one is in a rush about it, so least of all should the patient be.

A factor that is never talked about is finance. Patients, providers, state or insurers, and the myriad others involved with prostate cancer. (See quote at the front of this book.) I am in no position to give an analysis of multiple-payer systems, but the UK single-payer system, in its current iteration, has potential barriers to the implementation of a rational form of treatment, even though active surveillance has been received well here, and an analysis some years ago (2010) showed that 39% of men were on active surveillance protocols.

The difficulty in the UK Health Service in its current iteration is that despite a closed budget elements are trying to 'make money', which inevitably means that someone else will have a net loss. Modern surgical equipment is expensive, especially robotics, and trusts (the managing part of what used to be called hospitals) need an identifiable 'funding stream'. Should less prostate surgery be performed or radiation given, almost certainly less of a problem as there will always be other tumours to take up the slack, pressure could be exerted on patients to accept treatments they may not benefit from, and on clinicians 'to keep up their numbers'. UK patients may be significantly cut adrift from similar high-income countries by its inability to be flexible, which paradoxically in a closed financial system should be very easy.

It is, perhaps, a short diversion to consider British changes in their health care system, and how this impacts on treating patients in which uncertainty is constant, evidence is frequently poor or non-existent, and people making decisions that directly influence how patients, or indeed which patients are treated, are increasingly taken by people with no medical training, and guidelines, and their imperfect understanding of what they mean, to assist their understanding. It is a curious system.

Rather than investing heavily in nurses, doctors and equipment, although some of this was done, the British adopted a method which may have owed much to the pre-Second World War theory of 'The Indirect Approach'. The NHS invested massively in managers, some with a medical background but most without. From fewer than a 1,000 senior managers in 1997, the NHS acquired just under 40,000 by 2010. It was difficult to see clearly what their role was, although existing systems of clinical firms, clinical secretaries with major administrative responsibilities were superseded by managerial methods untried in the health care context, or any other from what I can see, and some major episodes of patient mortality, such as the Mid-Staffordshire scandal, were associated with these. But it was the numbers rather than the inevitable and predictable outcomes that impressed long term. By 2010 in my own city there were 610 managers for 626 consultant clinicians. Only in the pre-Second World War Soviet Army appeared this ratio of managers (Commissars) to experts. The Soviet system was rapidly jettisoned with the catastrophic defeats in the summer of 1941, and the seminal victories of Stalingrad, Kursk and Byelorussia were fought with a conventional structure. It makes for an interesting comparison.

Three incidents of these effects on clinical practice, the last two prostate cancer-related, illustrate the tension in working conditions these structures brought about.

In 1976 cisplatin was shown to cure patients with non-seminomatous testis cancer. This is an uncommon disease but very distressing to manage, as virtually all the patients were young men, and previously many had not done well. In common with many UK units we had a simple way of care. Any young man found to have a lump in his testis was seen in the next clinic, either that afternoon, or the following morning. This enabled them and their family to be told exactly what was to happen. They were then admitted and put on the next list, either that afternoon or the following morning, as appropriate. They bumped down the list order every other case. The operation was not long and rarely led to any existing patient being cancelled. All their bloods had been done prior to the operation, and their imaging was done the following day once they were comfortable. They were then booked into the oncologist's clinic the following week when all results were available, and the *necessary treatment often commenced that same day, time in this particular cancer being at a premium. You can imagine my distress to find a young man of 17 had been sent home by the admissions system because the target for urgent cases was two weeks, and in order to comply with this standard, the patient had received a date two weeks hence instead. There was an earnest hope that a bed would be available. When it was succinctly pointed out that these tumours could double in size in two weeks and they could well be looking at a young man who now had every chance of cure being unsalvageable two weeks down the line, the old system was reactivated, but ever since each case is a constant and individual battle; you cannot fight seven days a week, indefinitely.*

The second was more relevant to a prostate cancer patient. As has been explained most patients received their ADT by use of LHRH injections but a few still elected to have an orchidectomy to avoid 'all the bother of injections'. The patients in this category had progressive or symptomatic metastases and were always listed as urgent. To my distress, again, I found the patient had been bounced out of his bed by a patient requiring a minor procedure who had been waiting quite a long time. It was explained to me that there was now a traffic light system in place, which I thought was fine, until I learnt that patients who were an administrative problem, having missed their target date for their procedure, were being brought in as 'red light cases' and bouncing genuine urgent cases. We then told our patient to come to A & E department, thus completely abusing the system, in the patient's best interests.

The last, and probably most worrying of all in how it defines the new culture that has been imported, occurred during a morning's outpatient clinic. I was asked to go to the phone by someone who would not give their name but insisted on talking to me personally. This was an administrator from one of our neighbouring teaching centres, with which, as departments we had carried out a lot of collaborative work. Would I speak to the Chief Executive? I asked then to call back in five minutes and finished talking to the patient with me and took the call in the consulting room rather than the corridor.

Right, he said, we have had 24 deaths from prostate cancer in our hospital in the last month. We are measured against you lot, and you have had none. What are they doing up here? I explained that we only very rarely had patients with prostate cancer die in our hospital, because we had two excellent hospices in the city; the disease, even in its terminal stage, was still comparatively slow, so there was usually ample time to get such patients into the appropriate hands of the hospice doctors and nurses, so that specialist end of life care was available to them. I said my colleagues there, many of whom were friends, did exactly the same as we did, not least because both units put large numbers of patients into clinical trials. Surely you do the same as us? Well, he said, the first hospice here is just about to open. Well, I said, that is surely your answer. All these patients are receiving end of life care in hospital, and this will soon change. The phone was put down.

Later I heard from my friend who was Clinical Lead at the time. He had been ambushed in the car park when arriving at ten to eight, and taken to a meeting of the Trust Board, presented with this information, told about our comparator, and asked why they were killing all these patients. He is a tough and robust guy, but he said he was just stunned and could only babble (his words) that we were just like them and did nothing different. This case was obviously resolved rapidly, but without any apology, but the culture of blame and being guilty until innocence is proven does go against the conventions of what people assume to be a very central British value.

It is also easy to understand the distress of doctors who receive letters from the General Medical Council (GMC), which concern matters they had assumed had been dealt with some time ago. The standard managerial operating procedure appears to open a local inquiry and at the same time report the doctor to the GMC. Very often the local matter is resolved within a couple of weeks, but the GMC's laborious processes always take in excess of six months. The effect on the doctor of receiving a letter to say they are being investigated for something they thought long since finished with is often startling and has led to unhappy consequences. Over a five-year period in the recent past, nearly 100 doctors before the GMC died suddenly, and the worry was that these were suicides. The GMC ordered an independent review by an eminent psychiatrist that found cases that were explicable because of illness, but a rump of a couple of dozen or so appeared directly attributable to the GMC process, giving them, as I unkindly remarked to a couple of their senior people, who in fairness have strenuously tried to improve the system, a higher mortality rate than any surgeon in the country.

What, therefore, can be done?

First, it is essential that people know and understand the natural history of prostate cancer. They must be aware of its length, and that identification of both high- and low-risk individuals is uncertain, but no action needs to be precipitous.

All benefits of any treatment are fifteen to twenty years hence; side effects that materially alter life are immediate. The effects of overdiagnosis and subsequent overtreatment must be acknowledged by all participants. Physicians must recognise that, currently, they cannot identify any man who will benefit from treatment unequivocally, nor guarantee that no side effects from treatment will ensue. They have to further accept that mass therapy has not reduced the underlying mortality of this cancer by more than the odd percentage point in forty years. Patients must have time to be observed; to see what their cancer is doing and understand their prospects over these very long timescales, their general health and what precisely they wish for themselves.

Secondly, for this to happen, prostate cancer support groups, prostate cancer-oriented charities and donors to research groups must have an understanding and a common acceptance of time and its slowness, so no decision should be rushed, and in this particular cancer, cancer survivors means surviving with or without complications of therapy, not being alive five or ten years after treatment, which is just what happens to men who have no treatment.

If the war analogy of 'fighting cancer', early therapy saves lives, is not acknowledged as not so in this cancer, then no progress will be made.

It is patently obvious that men at risk need to be identified and treated differently from those in which the cancer will do little harm in their lifetime. We can only do this by carefully monitoring all patients, developing new blood and tumour markers, and putting research funding into finding why somebody's tumour that looks the same as others by all means at our disposal currently, behaves very differently. This means that individualised medicine has to come about, and our research should be forcing this along.

Many men and their families in the end are persuaded by their physician's steer. Only if all those treating prostate cancer accept this, or produce irrefutable evidence to the contrary, which means proper trials and actual outcomes, not actuarial ones, will patients have the confidence to be monitored and accept a change in direction.

The results of the Johns Hopkins analysis of their retrospective surgical results, showing only a small group appeared to benefit from surgery, and for which Walsh designed his operation to the great benefit of many men, have been trialled for twenty years in real time. The death rate has not changed, the ability to deliver this procedure, even with robot-assisted surgery, is not as good as Walsh or some of the other pioneers, so that in 2018, significant continence problems affect up to 20% of patients, and erectile dysfunction over 50%. These side effects restricting the last quarter of men's lives need not occur on the scale that has happened in the last twenty-five or more years.

It is this lost life that needs to be given back, and it starts with the proverb, 'hasten slowly'. All cancers are different, and to paraphrase Tolstoy, all cancers are different in their own particular way. Mass side effects for the many, to gain perhaps some benefit for the few has been tried and has failed. Patients, to retrieve their lost lives, in prostate cancer need a different approach. Active surveillance will likely redress the balance for the many.

Patient R was a lady, so did not have prostate cancer but she did have metastatic breast cancer, and what happened to her I do not understand. She was admitted under the care of the Professorial Unit in a famous London teaching hospital, where I was a house surgeon (intern, foundation 1 doctor). Patient safety was of paramount concern in those days, so that all tiers of junior doctors had their time of appointment staggered, so that as in my case my fellow house surgeon had already done three months in the post. He had admitted patient R, and for the next seven or eight weeks she had been nursed in one of two side cubicles at the end of this conventional Nightingale ward, in the expectation that she would shortly die. He moved across and I had looked after her for four or five weeks when following the professorial ward round, we were never spoken to directly, but the orders came down to us through the grades that this patient was to go home. She had been bed bound all the time she was with us (and because this is not an exercise in starry-eyed nostalgia) but for all the time I had been on the firm, no one other than we housemen had seen and talked to her, and the entourage had merely swept past her cubicle.

She had been superbly nursed, so was well fed, had no bed sores, the Brompton cocktail she took meant that she said she had no pain, but just felt very weak. She had been consistently anaemic, with a HB of 9.0 all the time she had been in, but it had not dropped. The ward sister felt her family could take her and cope, and when I saw her and explained that it was thought she should go home, she was very happy with that de-cision. I discussed her with my colleague, and we agreed that she might feel better, and would certainly look better if we transfused her. So she had two units of blood and went home, departing on a stretcher.

Although there were no bone scans routinely then, x-rays of skull, chest, limbs, spine and pelvis had shown that everywhere was riddled with lytic secondaries.

Just before he left my colleague came up to the ward. He had just done an outpatient clinic, and Patient R had turned up. Not only turned up but walked in wearing a new coat and hat, and she said, feeling very well. There was no pain, she had out on a little weight, and she had not become anaemic again. He had given her another appointment just be-fore I left and hoped she would turn up.

And turn up she did. Still well, mobile, not anaemic, and no pain. I don't know what to do, I said to her. We could do some more x-rays, but we won't do anything unless they are painful. Why don't I discharge you? If things get worse, your doctor can always send you back. Well, she said, I'm not coming back to that dying room, so I'll just see how it goes.

I returned to the unit eighteen months later and tried to find out whether she had come back. She hadn't, but London is a big place and she could quite easily have been admitted terminally to any six hospitals in the relatively near vicinity, but I wonder, and have always wondered whatever it might have been in the blood that arrested at least this ram-paging tumour.

'There are more things in heaven and earth, Horatio, than was dreamt of in your philosophy.'

ABOUT THE AUTHOR

Qualified at UCH,London in 1971,and undertook surgical and urological training in Bristol, Oxford, and Leeds. Appointed Consultant Urological Surgeon in Leeds 1982.I have been active within my own hospital and was Chair of the Senior Medical Staff Committee during the new consultant negotiations. I was also Vice Dean of the Medical School for St. James.1987 – 1992.

I am a great supporter of BAUS and have served on Council and as Treasurer, during which latter period we set up the Director of Training post, and together with Mike Wallace, the Section of Oncology. I was part of the College 'rapid reaction team, and subsequently served as

a clinical assessor for the National Clinical Assessment Service (NCAS).I was also an assessor for appeals for the STA and then PMETB. I served as member and Treasurer of BUF subsequently UF.

My main research interest has been in collaborative clinical trials mostly concerned with urological cancer. I was a member of and then chaired the Yorkshire Urological cancer research

group (YUCRG), and was active in the MRC Urological cancer research group and its subcommittees on prostate, bladder and kidney; I chaired the MRC superficial bladder cancer committee. Latterly I have chaired the NCRI Bladder Studies group. I joined the EORTC-GU

group (European Organisation into the research and treatment of Cancer). I chaired the Prostate Cancer committee and the Quality Control committee and as contributing and leading a number of studies was part of the Global group that initiated the first co-operative study between American and European collaborative groups, this on intermittent hormone therapy for prostate cancer.

I have supported the EAU (European Association of Urology) been a member of its Board , and served with the European School of Urology, and the History of Urology section, as well as helping to set up the European Urological Oncology section. My main work in Europe has been with the European Board of Urology (EBU) which is responsible for regulatory affairs and the harmonization of urological training and assessment. It has a direct, although somewhat byzantine connection to the EU commission, and serves a similar purpose to the American Urological Board exams, against which it is calibrated, the FEBU exam has been developed to act as' a mark of excellence' not 'a license to practice', allowing individual states to determine licensing and credentialing, and whether additional tests of knowledge or competence are necessary. Several countries have incorporated the complete FEBU into their exit assessments, whilst many others have incorporated part, usually the written, into their exit assessments.

This year 261 candidates will take the oral exam and the hope is that more European states will use it. Interestingly the European residents in training voted two years ago to have the written exam only in English unless it was part of the national exit process. I was President of the EBU from2006-2008.

I retired from St James in 2008 but cotinued as a Commumity Urologist until 2018 doing outreach NHS diagnostic Clinics.I remain a member of the Oversight Committee for Urological trials but will probably stop at the end of this year (2019).

I have been a member of the BMA's DoctorsSupport Doctors team since 2012 acting aas an adviser to doctors on any topic they wish to choose,especially those who have been reported to the GMC.

I have been a school governor since 2013 and Chair of Governors for an East Leeds Primary school since 2016.

I was awarded an MA in Military History from Leeds University in 2009.

ABOUT THE PUBLISHER

L.R. Price Publications is dedicated to publishing books by unknown authors.

We use a mixture of both traditional and modern publishing options to bring our authors' words to the wider world.

We print, publish, distribute and market books in a variety of formats including paper and hardback, electronic books, digital audio books and online.

If you are an author interested in getting your book published, or a book retailer interested in selling our books, please contact us.

www.lrpricepublications.com

L.R. Price Publications Ltd,
27 Old Gloucester Street,
London, WC1N 3AX.
020 3051 9572
publishing@lrprice.com

Printed in Great Britain
by Amazon